BODY HARMONY

Copyright

BODY HARMONY

Balancing PCOS Through Nourishing Recipes: A Culinary Journey for Body Harmony

S.L. MILLS

Disclaimer

Disclaimer: General Food Safety Disclaimer

The reader assumes full responsibility for using their best judgment when cooking with raw ingredients such as beef, poultry, or eggs, and seeking information from an official food safety authority if they are unsure.

The reader must also take care to not physically injure themselves by coming into contact with hot surfaces, sharp blades, and other kitchen hazards.

It is the responsibility of the reader to review all listed ingredients in a recipe before cooking to ensure that none of the ingredients may cause a potential adverse reactions.

About me

I work in the healthcare field as an educator. I love great food and I found that the right foods can help bring a balance to our physical, mental and emotional well being. Our hormones and their impact on us as women can not be underestimated. This book is a labor of love for me. Polycystic ovarian syndrome has touched someone I hold very precious in my life and it inspired me to provide good, comforting meals that could help with managing good diet. I wanted to create recipes that not only would be flavorful but healthy as well.

TABLE OF CONTENTS

BREAKFAST

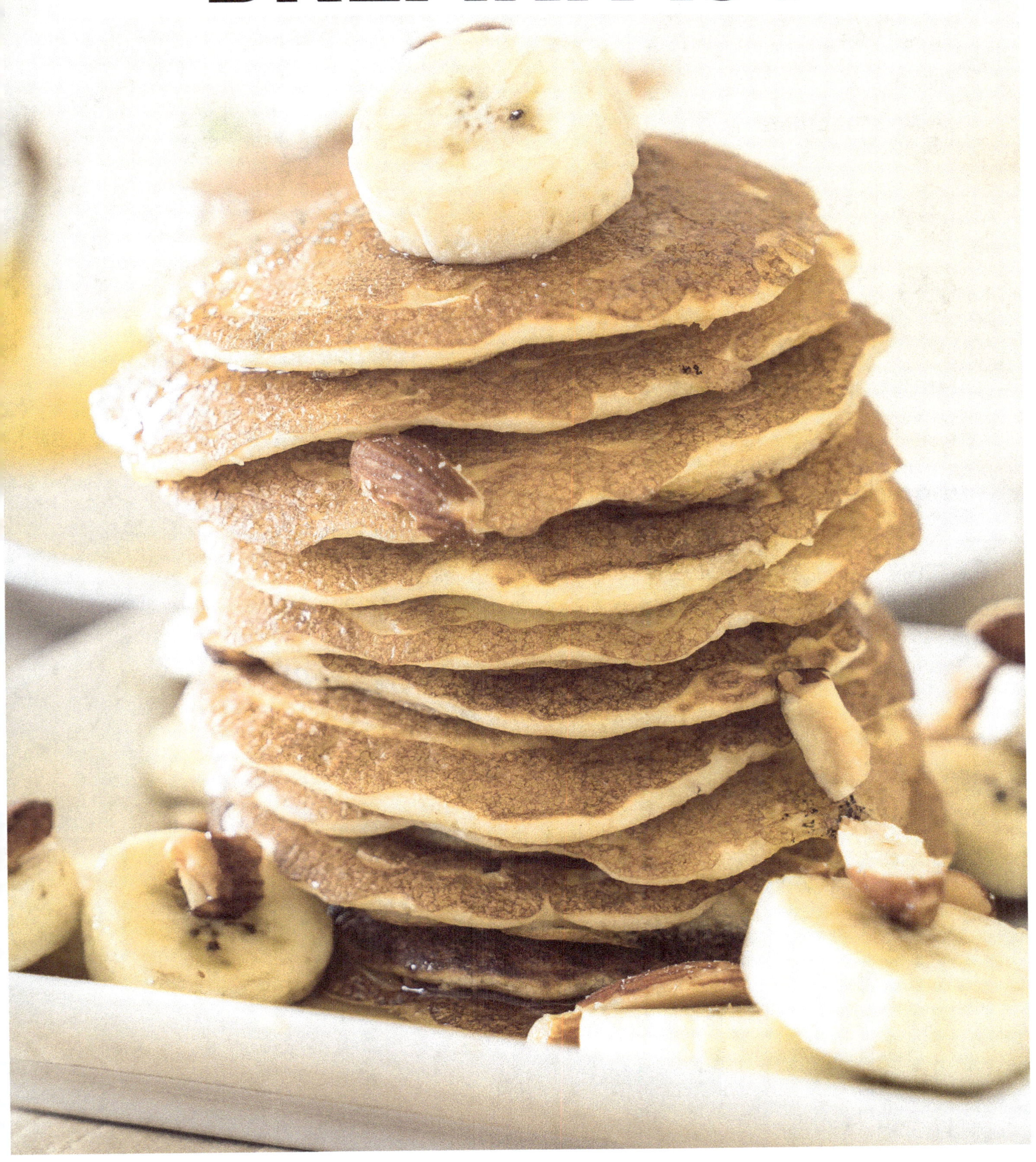

BERRY ALMOND SMOOTHIE BOWL

 **Prep time**
10 Min

 **Cook Time**
10 Min

 **Servings**
1

Nutrition Information

Calories: 325   Carbs: 35g
Protein: 8g   Fats: 18g

Ingredients

- 1 cup mixed berries (blueberries, strawberries, raspberries)
- 2 tbsp almond butter
- 1/2 cup almond milk
- 1 tbsp chia seeds
- 1 tbsp honey (optional)

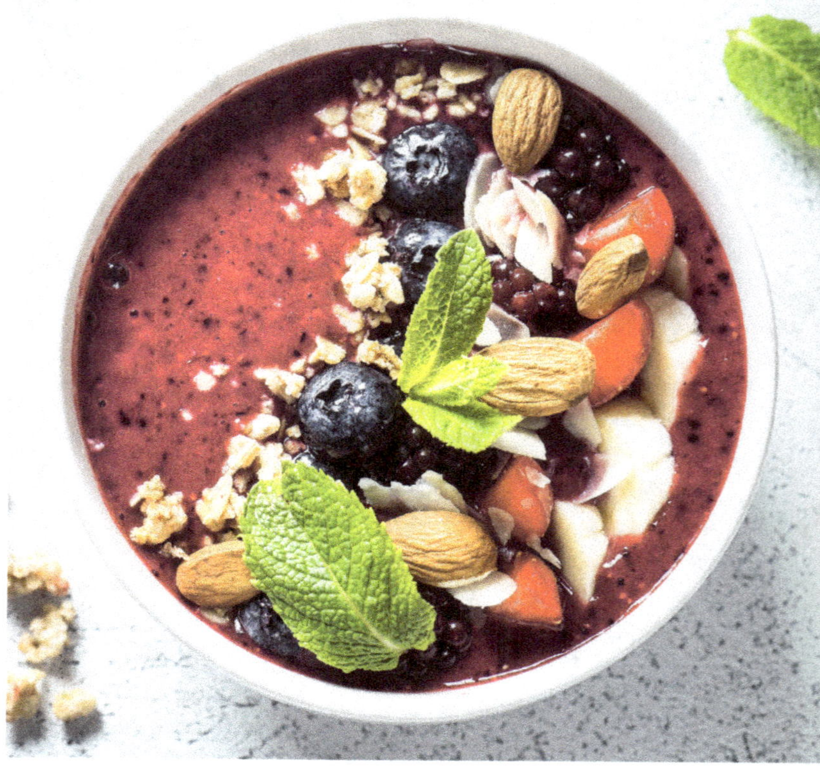

Directions

1. In a blender, combine the mixed berries, almond butter, almond milk, and honey (if using).
2. Blend until smooth.
3. Sprinkle chia seeds on top of the smoothie after pouring it into a bowl.
4. Add additional toppings if desired.

QUINOA AND SPINACH SCRAMBLE

 **Prep time**
10 Min

 **Cook Time**
10 Min

 **Servings**
2

Nutrition Information

Calories: 270   Carbs: 20g
Protein: 12g   Fats: 14g

Ingredients

- 1/2 cup cooked quinoa
- 1 cup spinach, chopped
- Four eggs
- 2 tbsp olive oil
- Salt and pepper to taste

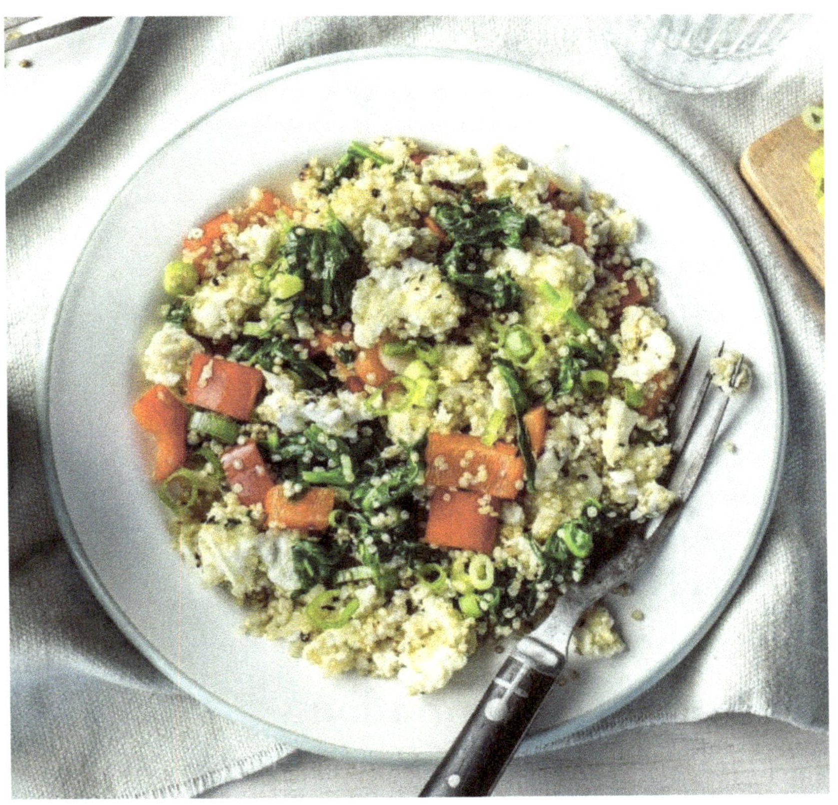

Directions

1. In a pan, warm olive oil over medium heat.
2. Add spinach and sauté until wilted.
3. Combine eggs, salt, and pepper using a bowl and whisk thoroughly.
4. Pour the eggs over the spinach and stir continuously.
5. Once the eggs begin to set, add the quinoa and stir until combined and cooked.

CHIA SEED & RASPBERRY OVERNIGHT OATS

Prep time
10 Min

Cook Time
0 Min

Servings
1

Nutrition Information

Calories: 280

Carbs: 40g

Protein: 7g

Fats: 8g

Ingredients

- 1/2 cup rolled oats
- 1 tbsp chia seeds
- 3/4 cup almond milk
- 1/2 cup raspberries
- 1 tbsp honey

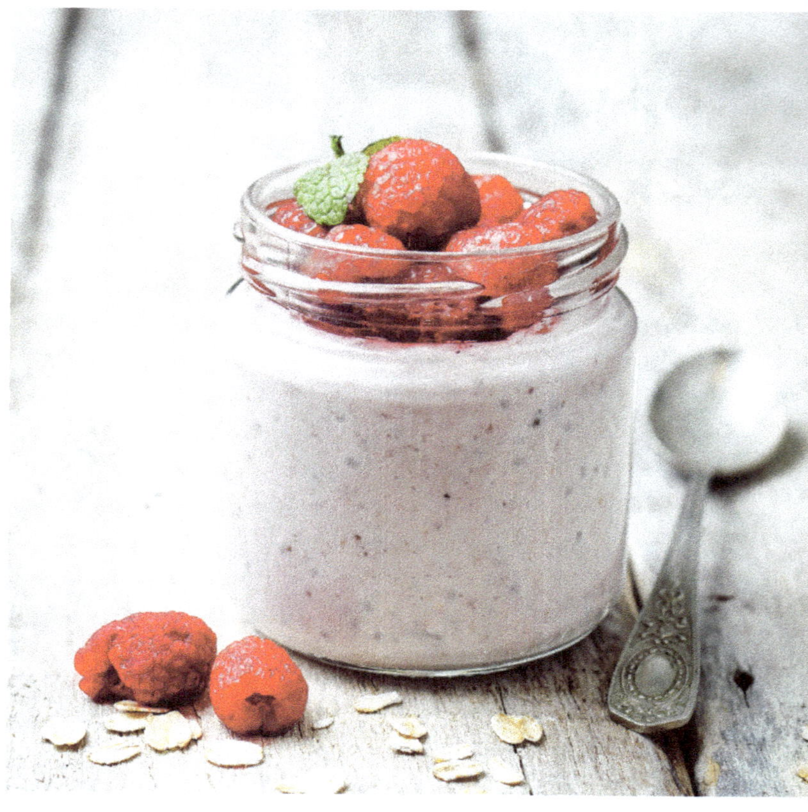

Directions

1. Combine the rolled oats, chia seeds, and almond milk in a jar or bowl.
2. Top with raspberries and drizzle with honey.
3. Cover and refrigerate overnight.
4. Before eating, stir well and add extra milk if desired.

GREEN DETOX SMOOTHIE

 **Prep time**
10 Min

 **Cook Time**
0 Min

 **Servings**
1

Nutrition Information

Calories: 110 Carbs: 28g
Protein: 2g Fats: 0.5g

Ingredients

- 1 cup spinach
- 1/2 cucumber
- 1 apple, cored and sliced
- 1/2 lemon, juiced
- 1 cup water

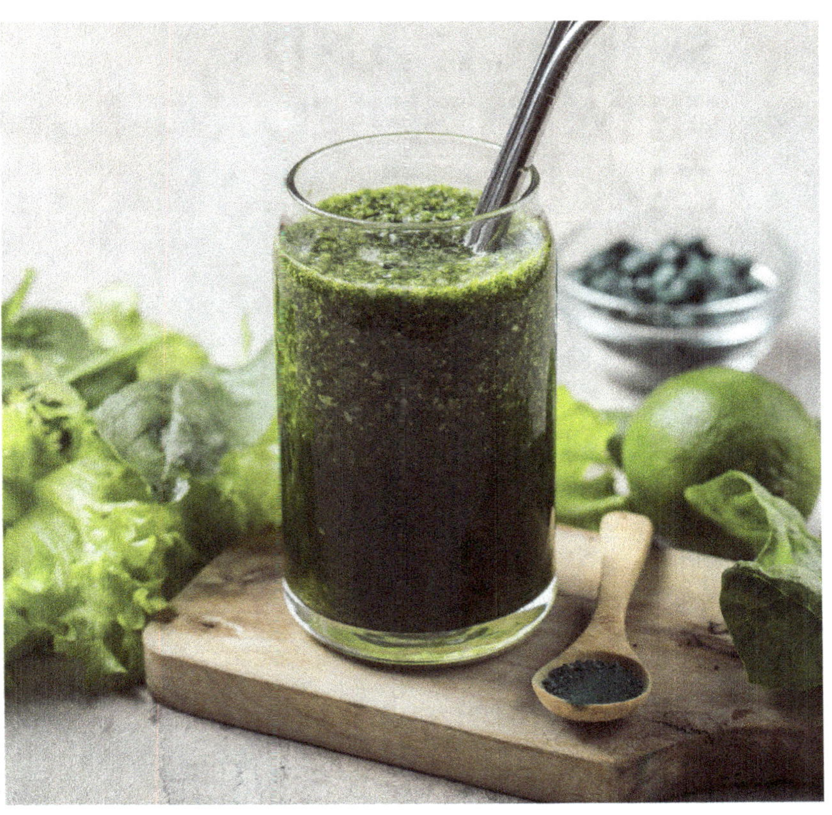

Directions

1. In a blender, combine all the ingredients.
2. Blend until smooth and creamy.
3. Pour into a glass and enjoy!

SPINACH AND FETA STUFFED OMELETTE

Prep time
10 Min

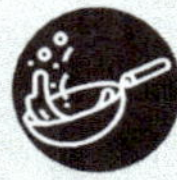

Cook Time
10 Min

Servings
1

Nutrition Information

Calories: 290
Protein: 20g

Carbs: 3g
Fats: 22g

Ingredients

- 3 eggs
- 1/4 cup feta cheese, crumbled
- 1/2 cup spinach, chopped
- 1 tbsp olive oil
- Salt and pepper to taste

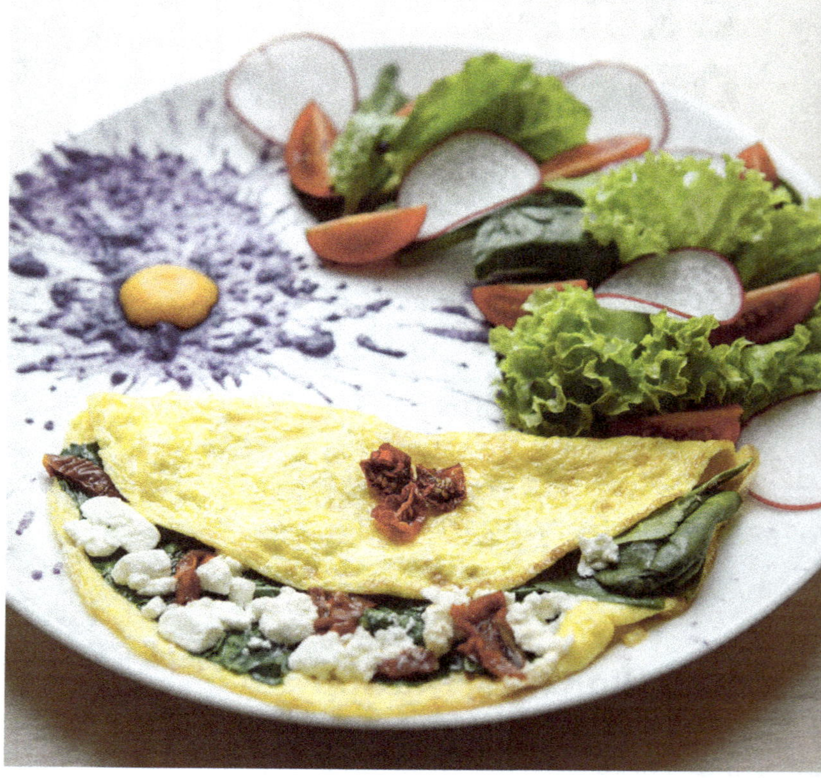

Directions

1. Mix some eggs, salt, and pepper in a bowl using a whisk.
2. Begin by warming olive oil in a pan over medium heat. Once heated, add spinach and sauté until it is fully wilted.
3. Pour the eggs over the spinach.
4. Once the edges start setting, sprinkle feta cheese on one half.
5. Once fully set, fold the omelet over the cheese and serve.

ALMOND BUTTER AND BANANA PANCAKES

 **Prep time**
10 Min

 **Cook Time**
10 Min

 **Servings**
2

Nutrition Information

Calories: 270   Carbs: 32g
Protein: 10g   Fats: 12g

Ingredients

- 2 ripe bananas, mashed
- 2 eggs
- 1 tbsp almond butter
- 1/4 tsp baking powder (gluten-free)
- Pinch of salt

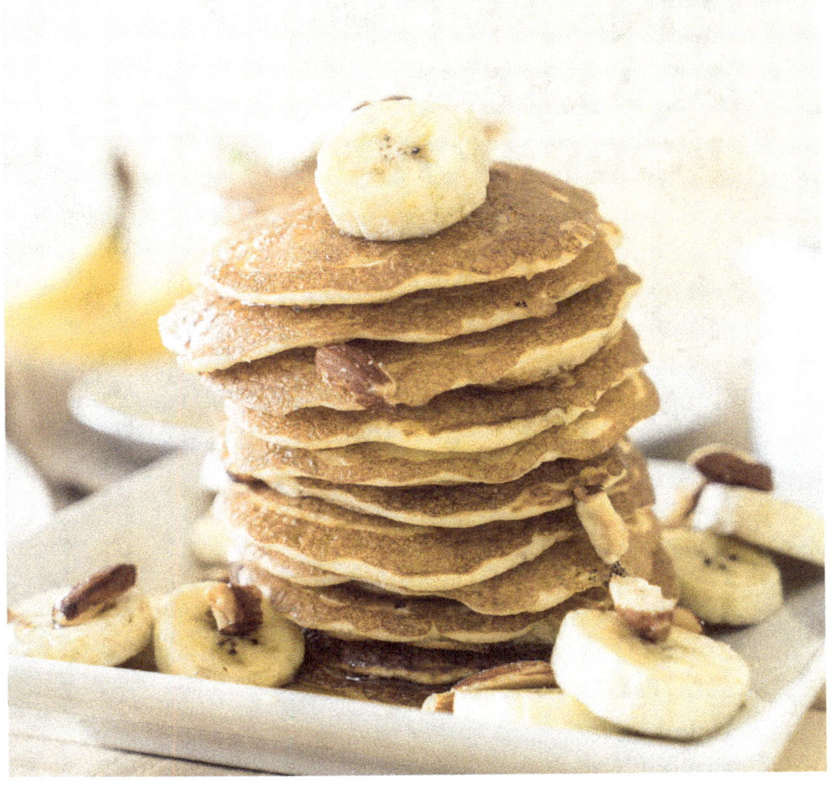

Directions

1. Combine mashed bananas, eggs, almond butter, baking powder, and salt in a mixing bowl.
2. Heat a non-stick skillet over medium heat.
3. Drop batter by 1/4 cup onto the skillet.
4. Prepare until bubbles form on the top, then flip and cook until browned on the other side.
5. Serve warm.

CINNAMON FLAXSEED PORRIDGE

Prep time
2 Min

Cook Time
5 Min

Servings
1

Nutrition Information

Calories: 180
Protein: 5g

Carbs: 12g
Fats: 12g

Ingredients

- 2 tbsp ground flaxseed
- 1 cup almond milk
- 1/2 tsp cinnamon
- 1 tbsp maple syrup or honey

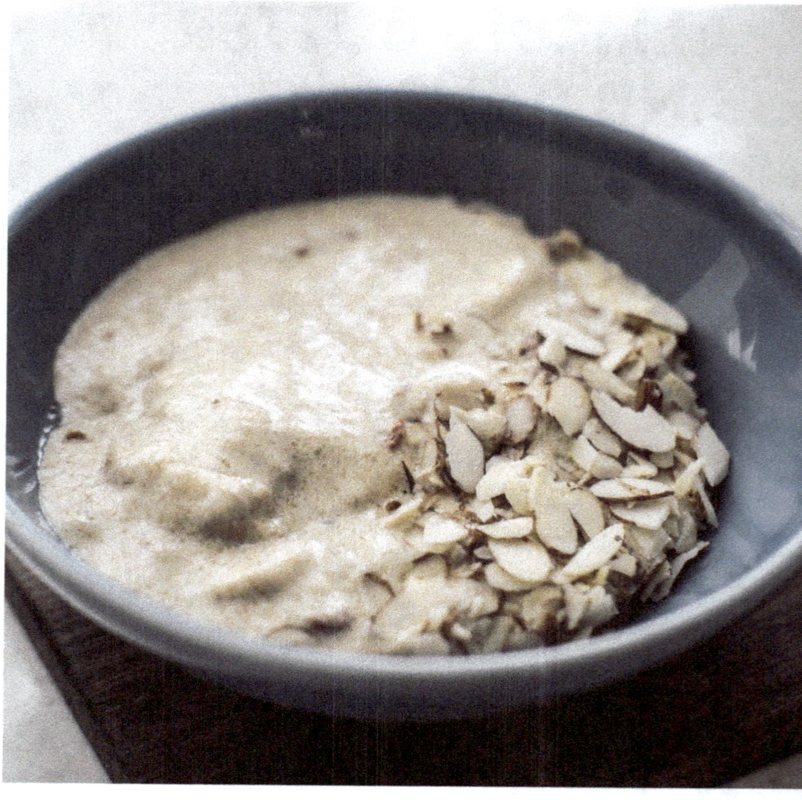

Directions

1. In a small-sized saucepan, bring almond milk to a low boil.
2. Stir in ground flaxseed and cinnamon.
3. Reduce heat and simmer until thickened.
4. Sweeten with maple syrup or honey. Serve warm.

BERRY NUT BREAKFAST PARFAIT

Prep time
10 Min

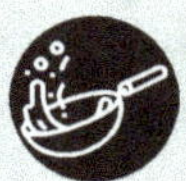

Cook Time
0 Min

Servings
1

Nutrition Information

Calories: 300   Carbs: 25g
Protein: 15g   Fats: 15g

Ingredients

- 1 cup Greek yogurt
- 1/2 cup mixed berries
- 1/4 cup mixed nuts (almonds, walnuts)
- 1 tbsp honey

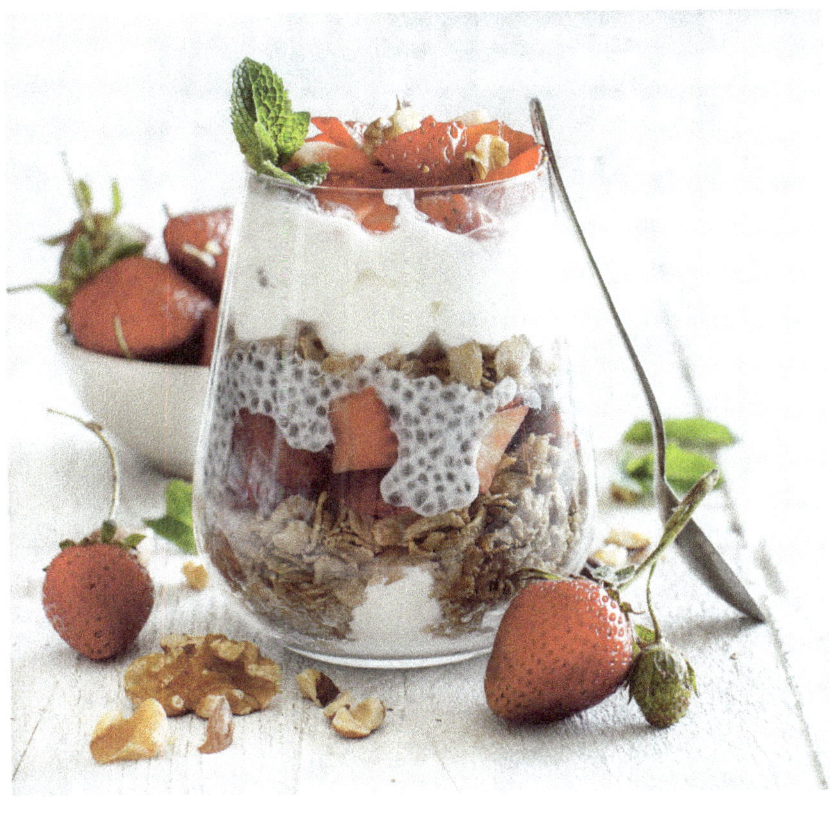

Directions

1. In a glass jar, layer Greek yogurt, berries, and nuts.
2. Drizzle honey over the top layer.
3. Repeat until all ingredients are used up. Serve immediately.

AVOCADO AND EGG BREAKFAST SANDWICH

Prep time
10 Min

Cook Time
10 Min

Servings
1

Nutrition Information

Calories: 370   Carbs: 30g
Protein: 14g   Fats: 23g

Ingredients

- 1 whole-grain English muffin
- 1/2 ripe avocado, sliced
- 1 egg
- 1 tbsp olive oil
- Salt and pepper to taste

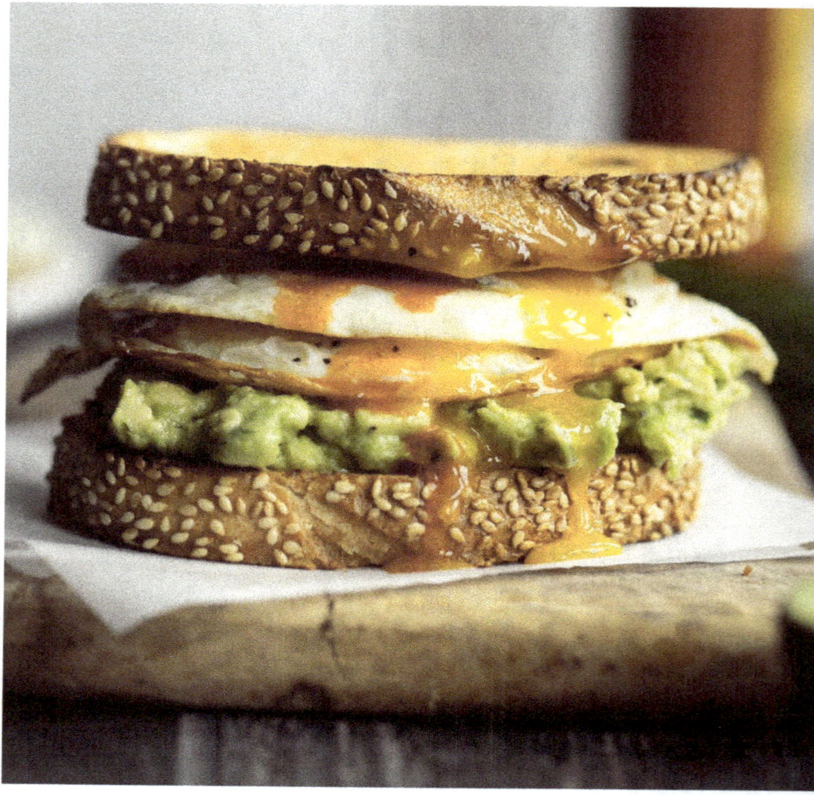

Directions

1. Toast the English muffin.
2. In a skillet, it is warming olive oil over medium heat. Crack the egg into the skillet.
3. Cook the egg to your liking (over-easy, sunny-side up, etc.).
4. Assemble the sandwich by placing avocado slices on one half of the muffin, followed by the egg, and then the other half of the muffin—season with salt and pepper.

COCONUT AND ALMOND MUFFINS (SUGAR-FREE)

Prep time
15 Min

Cook Time
20 Min

Servings
6 Muffins

Nutrition Information

Calories: 220
Protein: 7g

Carbs: 8g
Fats: 18g

Ingredients

- 1 cup almond flour
- 1/2 cup shredded coconut
- 3 eggs
- 1/4 cup coconut oil, melted
- 1 tsp baking powder
- Stevia or monk fruit to taste

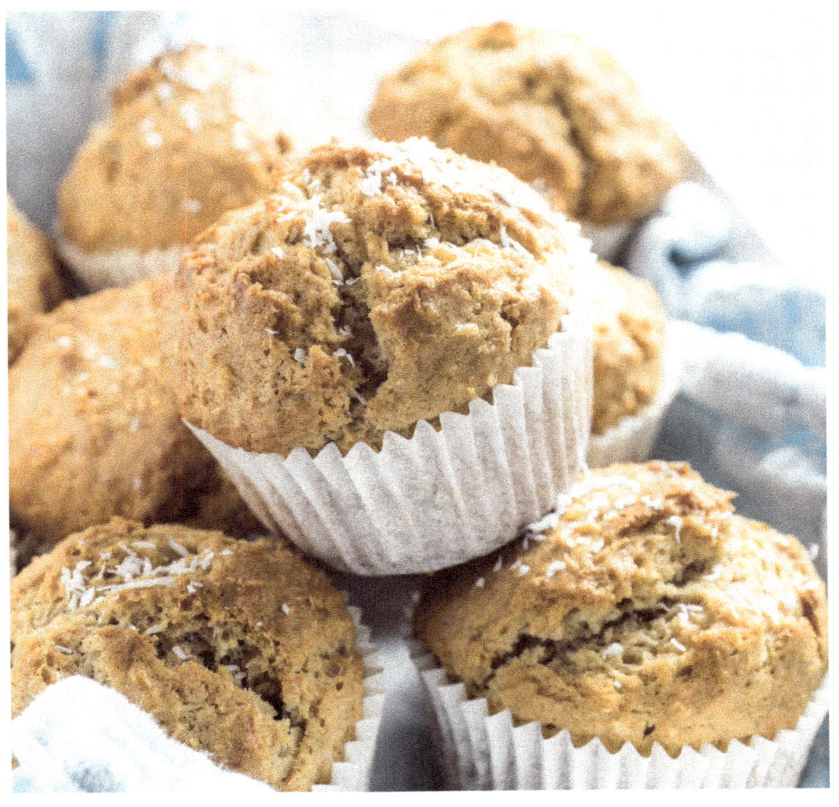

Directions

1. Preheat oven to 350°F (175°C).
2. Combine almond flour, shredded coconut, and baking powder in a bowl.
3. Stir in eggs, melted coconut oil, and sweetener.
4. Divide the mixture among 6 muffin cups.
5. Bake for 20 minutes or until the tip of a toothpick comes out clean.

LUNCH

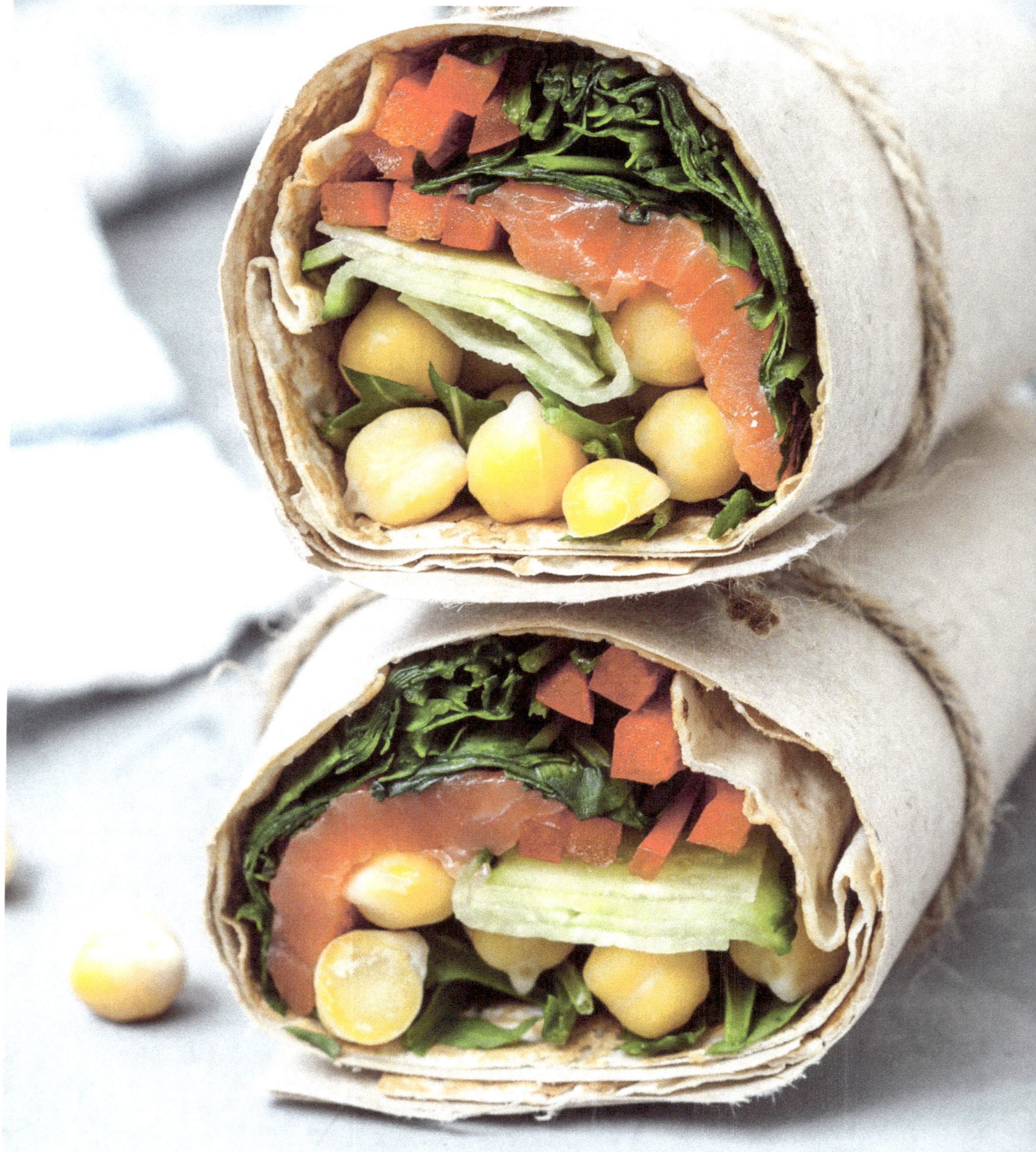

GRILLED LEMON HERB CHICKEN SALAD

Prep time
15 Min

Cook Time
15 Min

Servings
4

Nutrition Information

Calories: 270   Carbs: 8g
Protein: 30g   Fats: 12g

Ingredients

- 4 chicken breasts
- 2 lemons, juiced
- 2 tbsp olive oil
- 1 tbsp mixed dried herbs (thyme, oregano, rosemary)
- 4 cups mixed salad greens
- 1 cup cherry tomatoes, halved
- 1/2 red onion, thinly sliced
- 1/4 cup feta cheese
- Salt and pepper to taste

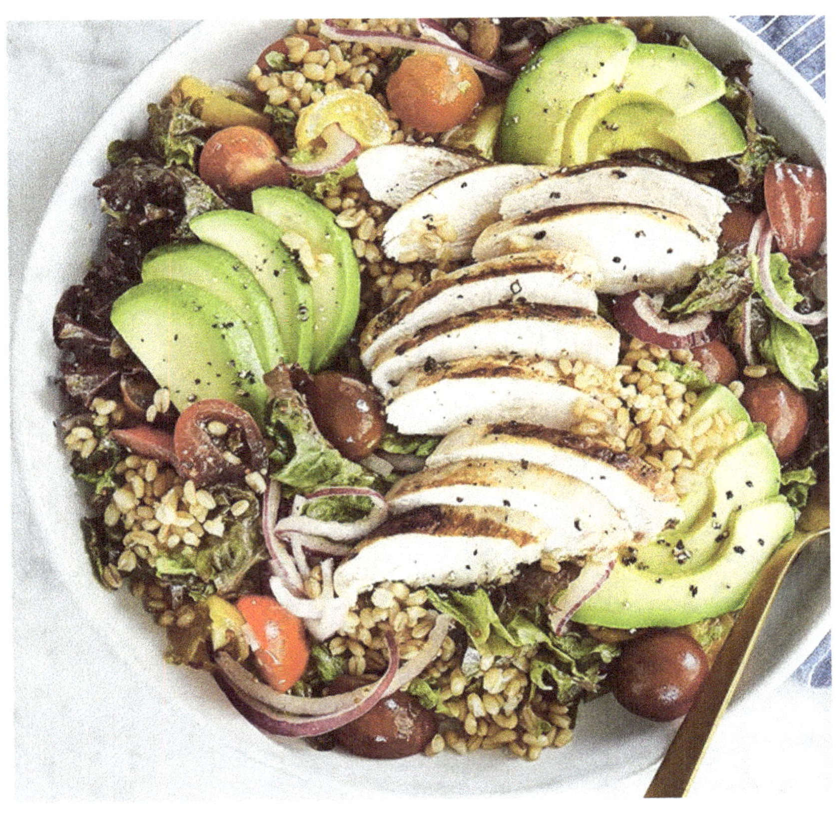

Directions

1. Whisk together lemon juice, olive oil, herbs, salt, and pepper in a mixing bowl.
2. Add chicken breasts to the mixture, ensuring they're well coated. Marinate for at least 30 minutes in the refrigerator.
3. Set a grill or grill pan over medium heat. After heating the grill, put the chicken breasts on it and cook each side for approximately 6-7 minutes or until thoroughly cooked.
4. Combine salad greens, cherry tomatoes, and sliced red onion in a large bowl.
5. Take the grilled chicken and cut it into bite-sized pieces. Then, add the chicken to the salad bowl. Sprinkle with feta cheese and toss lightly to combine.
6. Serve with your favorite dressing on the side.

SPINACH AND QUINOA POWER BOWL

Prep time
10 Min

Cook Time
20 Min

Servings
2

Nutrition Information

Calories: 320
Protein: 8g

Carbs: 38g
Fats: 16g

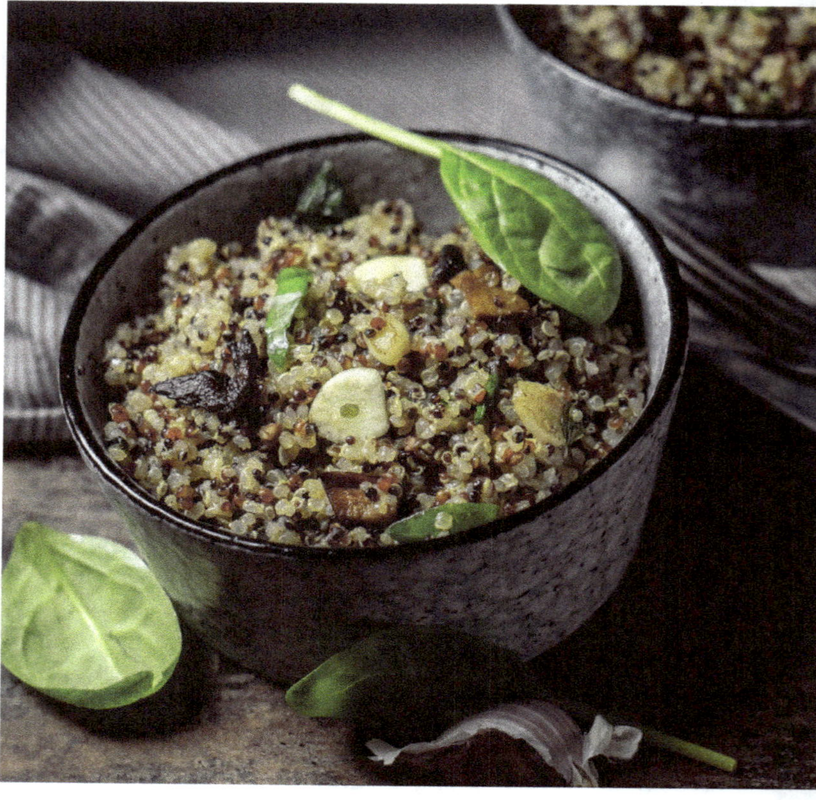

Ingredients

- 1 cup cooked quinoa
- 2 cups fresh spinach, washed and dried
- 1 avocado, peeled and sliced
- 1/2 cup cherry tomatoes, halved
- 2 tbsp pumpkin seeds
- 1 tbsp olive oil
- Salt and pepper to taste

Directions

1. Prepare quinoa according to package instructions. After cooking, use a fork to separate the grains and let them cool down.
2. Combine spinach, cooled quinoa, avocado slices, and halved cherry tomatoes in a large mixing bowl.
3. Just sprinkle some oil and a dash of salt & pepper to add flavor to the coat.
4. Toss the ingredients gently to combine. Garnish with pumpkin seeds before serving.

CHICKPEA AND VEGGIE WRAP

Prep time
15 Min

Cook Time
0 Min

Servings
2

Nutrition Information

Calories: 280   Carbs: 45g
Protein: 12g   Fats: 7g

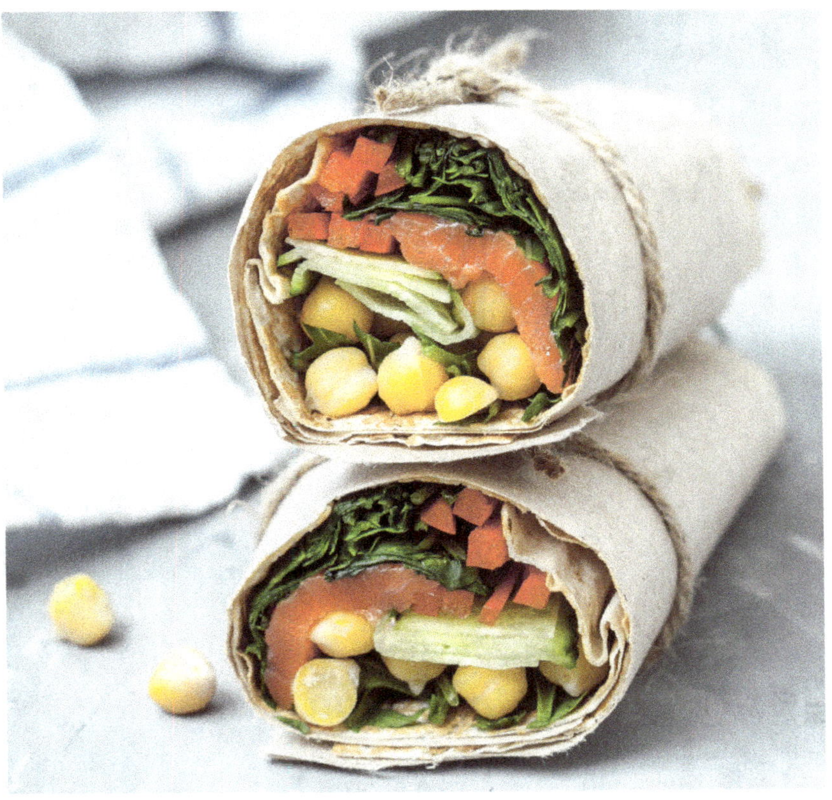

Ingredients

- 1 cup canned chickpeas, rinsed and drained
- 2 whole grain tortillas
- 1/2 cup shredded carrot
- 1/2 cucumber, thinly sliced
- 1/2 bell pepper, thinly sliced
- 2 tbsp hummus
- Salt and pepper to taste

Directions

1. Lay out the tortillas flat on a clean surface. Evenly spread hummus on each.
2. Scatter the chickpeas across the hummus-laden tortillas.
3. Arrange the shredded carrot, cucumber slices, and bell pepper evenly on top.
4. For seasoning, sprinkle a pinch of salt and pepper.
5. Roll each tortilla tightly, then slice in half diagonally for easier serving.

LENTIL SOUP WITH KALE

 **Prep time**
10 Min

 **Cook Time**
45 Min

 **Servings**
4

Nutrition Information

Calories: 220   Carbs: 32g
Protein: 14g   Fats: 5g

Ingredients

- 1 cup green lentils, rinsed and drained
- 4 cups vegetable broth
- 2 cups chopped kale, stems removed
- 1 medium onion, finely chopped
- 2 garlic cloves, minced
- 2 tbsp olive oil
- Salt and ground black pepper to taste

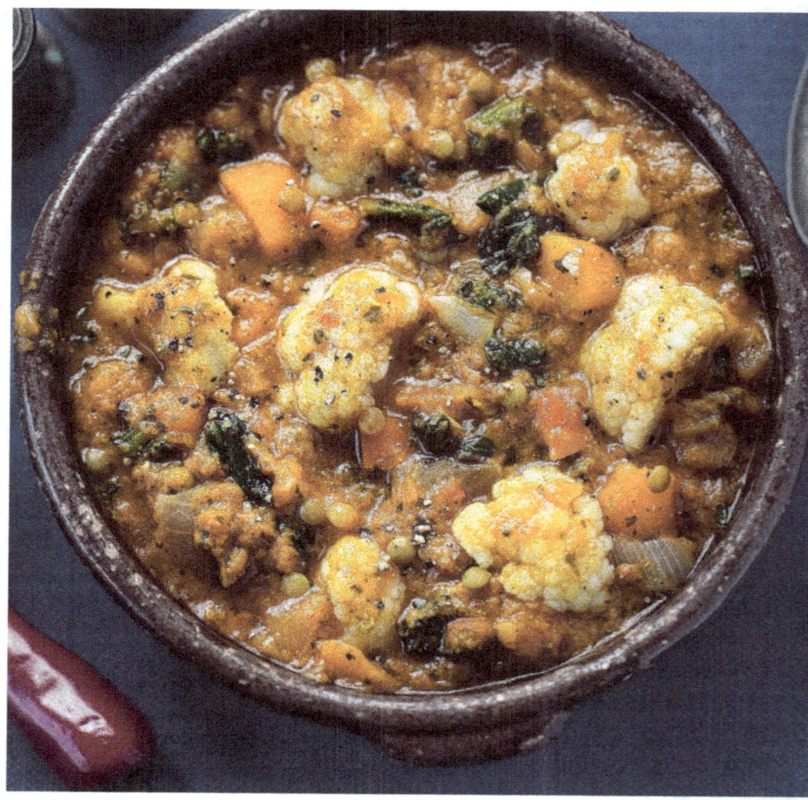

Directions

1. In a large-sized pot, warm the olive oil over medium heat. Add the chopped onion and sauté until translucent, about 3-4 minutes.
2. Add the minced garlic and prepare for 1-2 minutes, stirring occasionally.
3. Pour in the lentils and vegetable broth. Increase heat to high and bring to a boil.
4. After the water has come to a boil, turn the heat to a minimum and allow it to simmer for approximately 30 minutes or until the lentils have become tender.
5. Add the chopped kale and prepare for about 3 minutes until it is wilted.
6. Season your dish using salt and ground black pepper according to your taste. Serve the dish while it's still warm.

MEDITERRANEAN TUNA SALAD LETTUCE WRAPS

Prep time
15 Min

Cook Time
0 Min

Servings
2

Nutrition Information

Calories: 210   Carbs: 8g
Protein: 20g   Fats: 10g

Ingredients

- 1 can (150g) tuna in water, drained
- 1/2 cucumber, finely diced
- 1/2 bell pepper, finely diced
- 1/4 cup red onion, finely chopped
- 1/4 cup crumbled feta cheese
- 4-6 large lettuce leaves, washed and dried (like romaine or iceberg)
- 1 tbsp olive oil
- 1 tbsp fresh lemon juice
- Salt and ground black pepper to taste

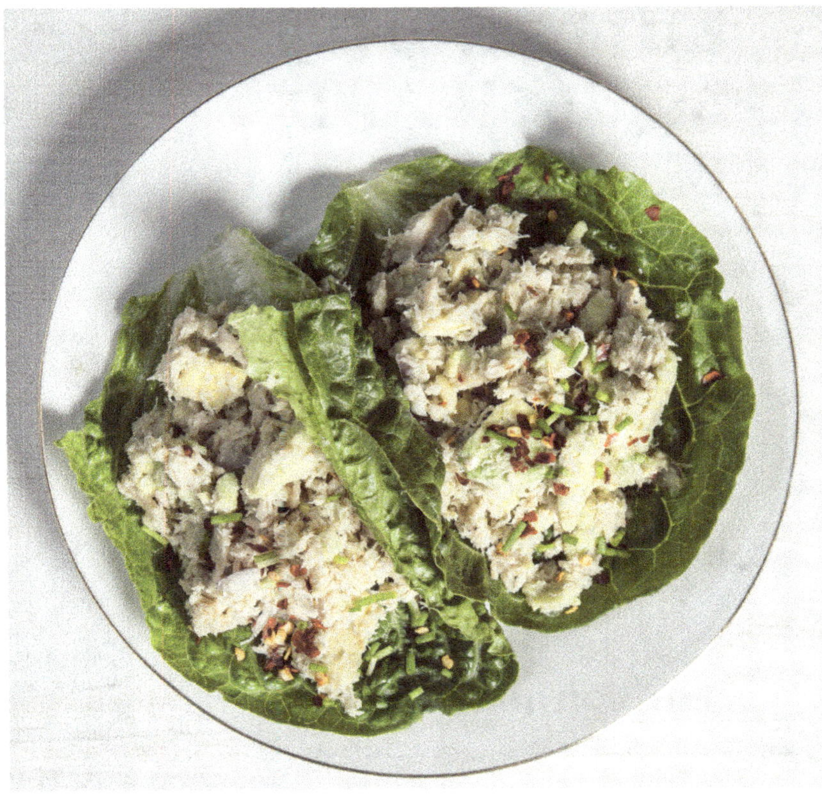

Directions

1. Combine the drained tuna, diced cucumber, bell pepper, chopped red onion, and feta cheese in a medium mixing bowl.
2. Mix the oil and lime juice in a small-sized bowl by whisking them. Drizzle this dressing over the tuna mixture, then gently stir to combine.
3. Mix blending with salt and ground black pepper, adjusting to your preference.
4. Scoop a generous amount of the tuna salad onto each lettuce leaf. Fold the lettuce around the filling and serve immediately.

BUTTERNUT SQUASH AND BLACK BEAN SALAD

 **Prep time**
20 Min

 **Cook Time**
25 Min

 **Servings**
3

Nutrition Information

Calories: 230　　Carbs: 36g
Protein: 7g　　Fats: 9g

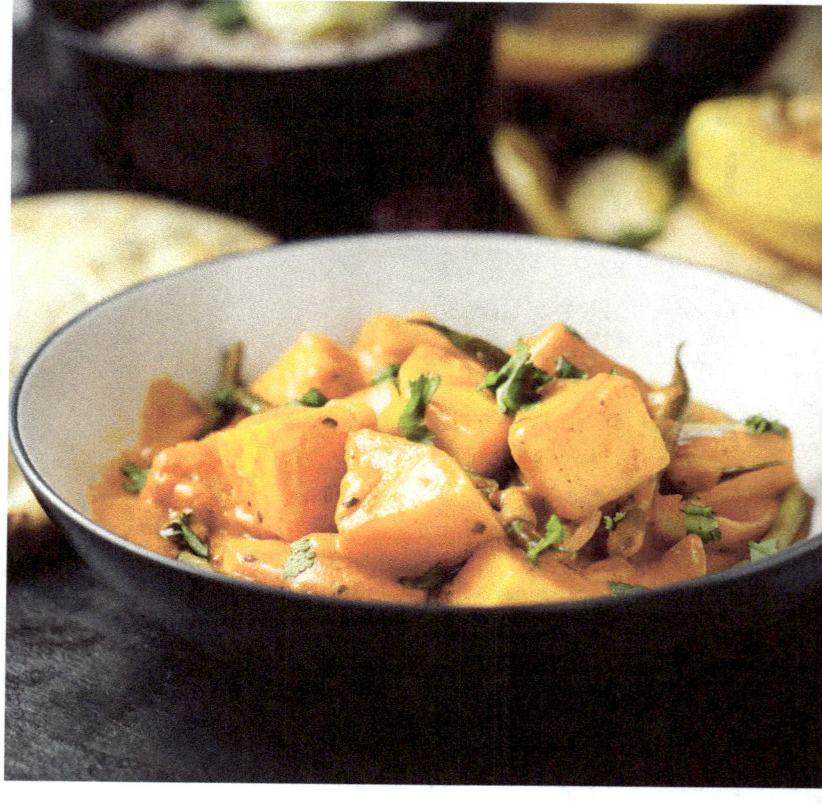

Ingredients

- 2 cups diced butternut squash
- 1 cup canned black beans, watered and drained
- 2 green onions, sliced
- 1/4 cup fresh cilantro, chopped
- 2 tbsp olive oil
- 1 tbsp lime juice
- Salt and ground black pepper to taste

Directions

1. Set your oven's temperature to 400°F (200°C). To prepare the butternut squash, lay it on a baking tray and sprinkle 1 tablespoon of olive oil. Add salt & pepper to taste, and then mix everything until the squash is evenly coated.
2. Roast the butternut squash in your oven for 20-25 minutes or until it gets tender and lightly browned. Remove from the oven and let it cool.
3. Combine the roasted butternut squash, black beans, green onions, and cilantro in a large-sized mixing bowl.
4. Drizzle the salad with the remaining oil and lime juice. Gently toss to combine. If required, add more salt and freshly ground black pepper to taste. You have the option of serving it either chilled or at room temperature.

CUCUMBER AND AVOCADO ROLL-UPS

 **Prep time**
15 Min

 **Cook Time**
0 Min

 **Servings**
2-3

Nutrition Information

Calories: 120   Carbs: 10g
Protein: 2g   Fats: 9g

Ingredients

- 1 large cucumber
- 1 ripe avocado, mashed
- 1/2 lemon, juiced
- 1 tbsp chopped fresh dill
- Salt and ground black pepper to taste

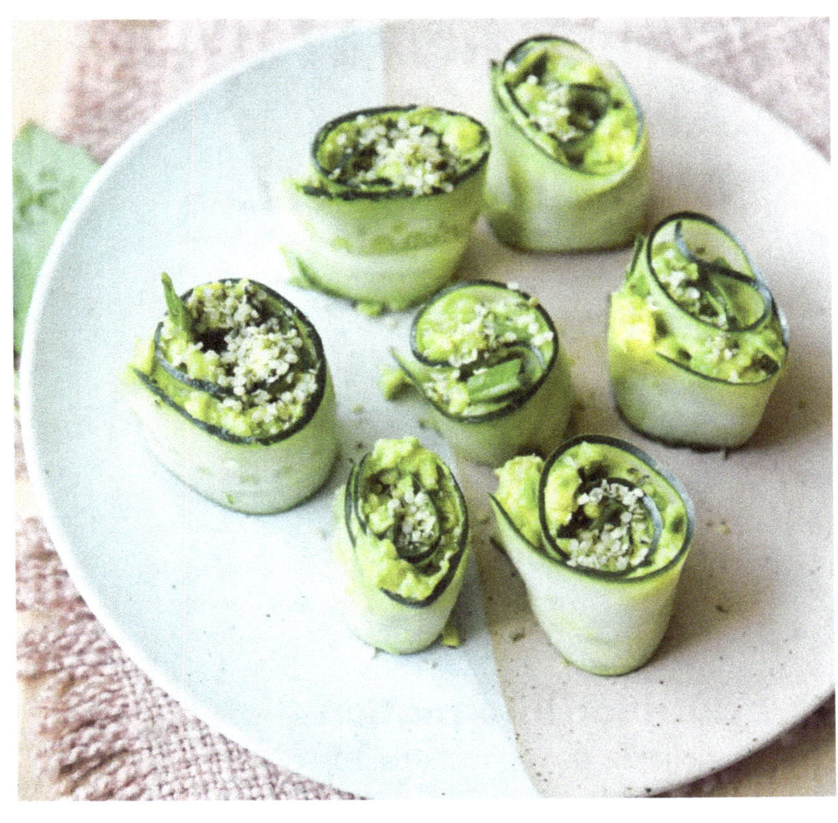

Directions

1. To create thin and long strips, utilize a vegetable peeler to slice the cucumber.
2. Combine the mashed avocado, lemon juice, and fresh dill in a mixing bowl. Season with salt and pepper to taste.
3. Lay out the cucumber strips and spread a small amount of the avocado mixture along each strip.
4. Carefully roll up each strip, securing it with a toothpick if needed. Serve immediately.

SWEET POTATO AND KALE BUDDHA BOWL

Prep time
20 Min

Cook Time
30 Min

Servings
2

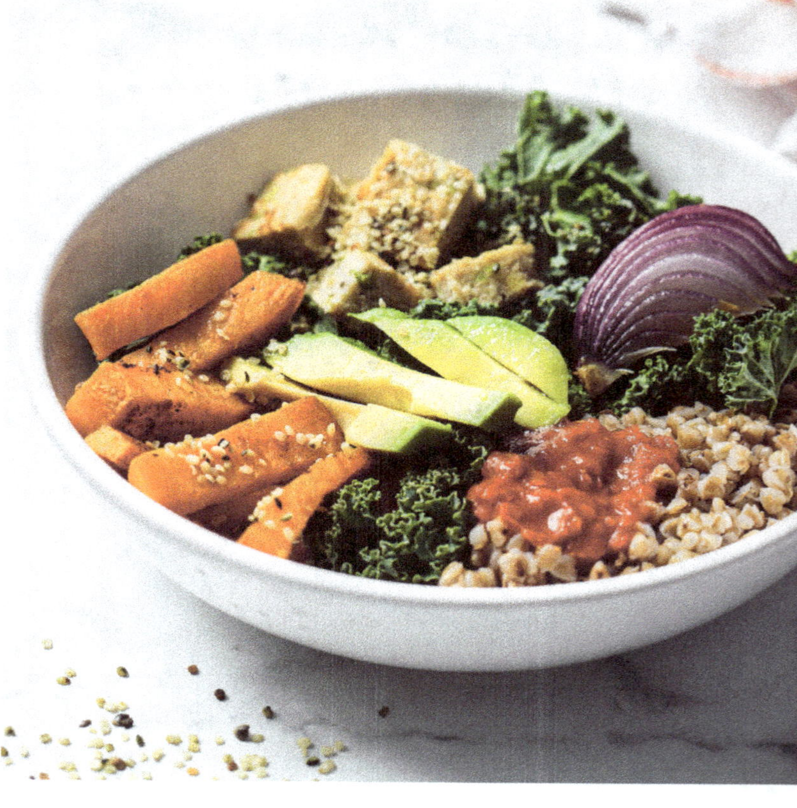

Nutrition Information

Calories: 270
Protein: 6g

Carbs: 50g
Fats: 6g

Ingredients

- 2 medium-sized sweet potatoes, cubed
- 2 cups kale, chopped
- 1/2 cup cooked quinoa
- 1 tbsp olive oil
- 1 tsp smoked paprika
- Salt and ground black pepper to taste

Directions

1. Adjust the oven's heat to 400°F (200°C). Mix sweet potato cubes with oil, smoked paprika, salt, & pepper in a bowl.
2. To prepare the sweet potato, spread the seasoned pieces on a cooking sheet and roast in the oven for around 25-30 minutes or until they become tender.
3. Layer cooked quinoa, roasted sweet potato, and chopped kale in a serving bowl.
4. Drizzle with your choice of dressing or a simple oil and lemon juice mix. Serve warm.

CAULIFLOWER FRIED RICE

Prep time
15 Min

Cook Time
15 Min

Servings
4

Nutrition Information

Calories: 140

Carbs: 18g

Protein: 8g

Fats: 5g

Ingredients

- 1 large head of cauliflower, riced
- 2 eggs, beaten
- 1 cup mixed vegetables (like peas, carrots, and corn)
- 2 green onions, chopped
- 2 tbsp soy sauce (low sodium)
- 1 tbsp sesame oil
- Salt and pepper to taste

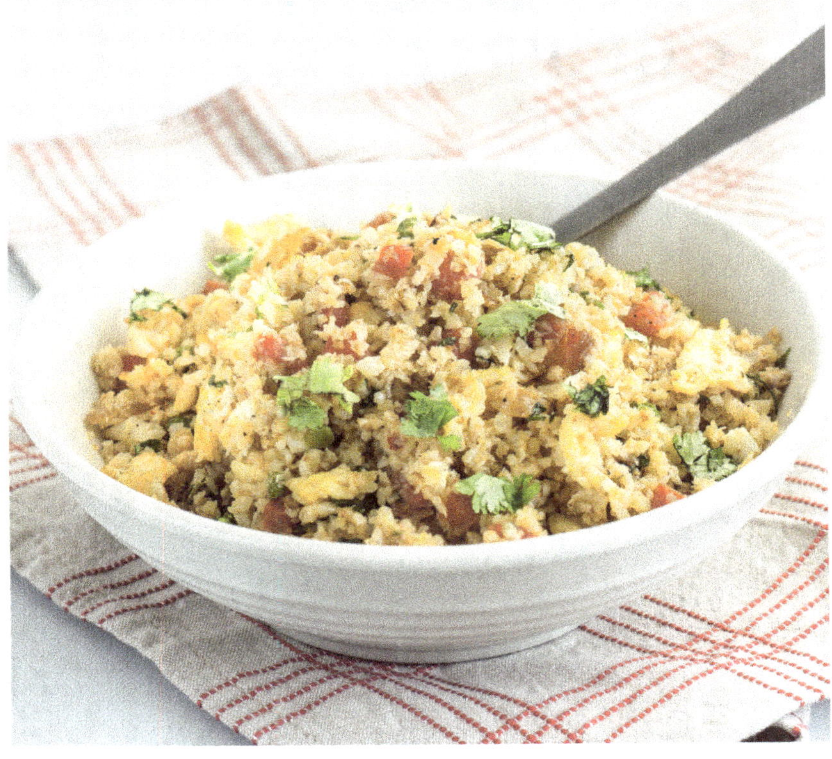

Directions

1. Warm the sesame oil over moderate-high heat in a large skillet or wok. Add the riced cauliflower and cook for 5-7 minutes or until slightly softened.
2. To prepare, first, move the cauliflower to one side of the pan. Then, pour the beaten eggs onto the opposite side. Scramble the eggs and combine them with the cauliflower.
3. Add the mixed vegetables and soy sauce. Stir to combine everything.
4. Continue cooking for another 5 minutes or until the vegetables are tender.
5. Garnish with chopped green onions before serving. Adjust seasoning if needed.

TURMERIC CHICKPEA SALAD

Prep time
15 Min

Cook Time
0 Min

Servings
3

Nutrition Information

Calories: 220   Carbs: 30g
Protein: 9g   Fats: 8g

Ingredients

- 1 can (15 oz.) chickpeas, drained and watered
- 1/2 cup red onion, finely chopped
- 1/4 cup fresh cilantro, chopped
- 1/2 tsp turmeric powder
- 1 tbsp olive oil
- 1 lemon, juiced
- Salt and ground black pepper to taste

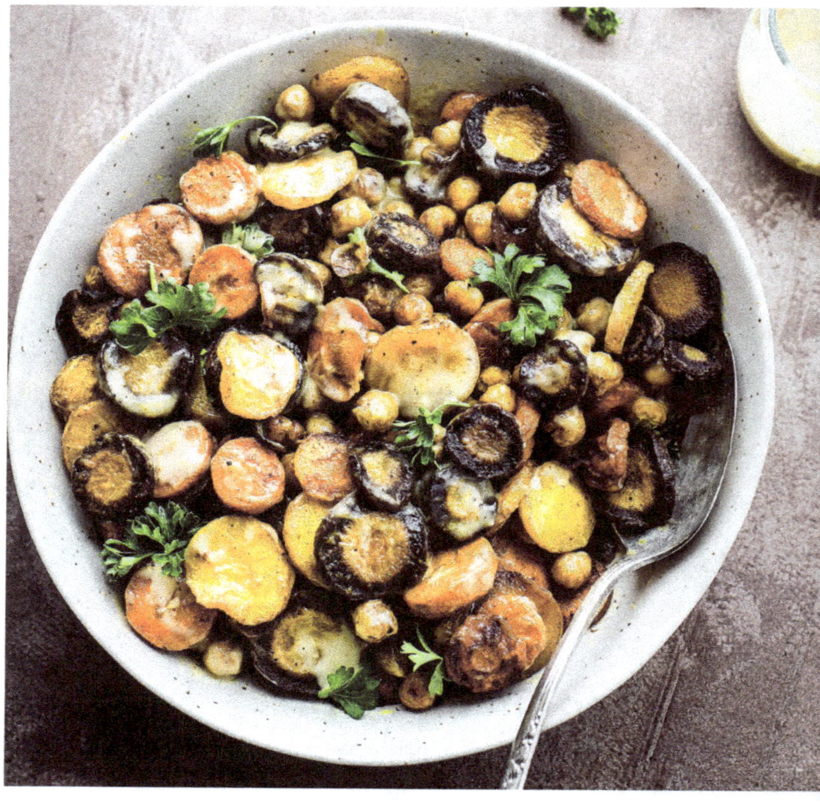

Directions

1. In a large bowl, combine chickpeas, red onion, and cilantro.
2. Whisk together olive oil, lemon juice, turmeric, salt, and pepper in a separate smaller bowl.
3. Mix the dressing with the chickpea mixture and stir thoroughly. Let it rest for 10 minutes before serving to allow the flavors to blend.

BROCCOLI AND CHEDDAR STUFFED PEPPERS

Prep time
15 Min

Cook Time
30 Min

Servings
4

Nutrition Information

Calories: 280   Carbs: 27g
Protein: 12g   Fats: 15g

Ingredients

- 4 large bell peppers, tops removed and seeds cleaned out
- 1 cup broccoli florets, finely chopped
- 1 cup cooked quinoa
- 1 cup cheddar cheese, shredded
- 2 tbsp olive oil
- Salt and ground black pepper to taste

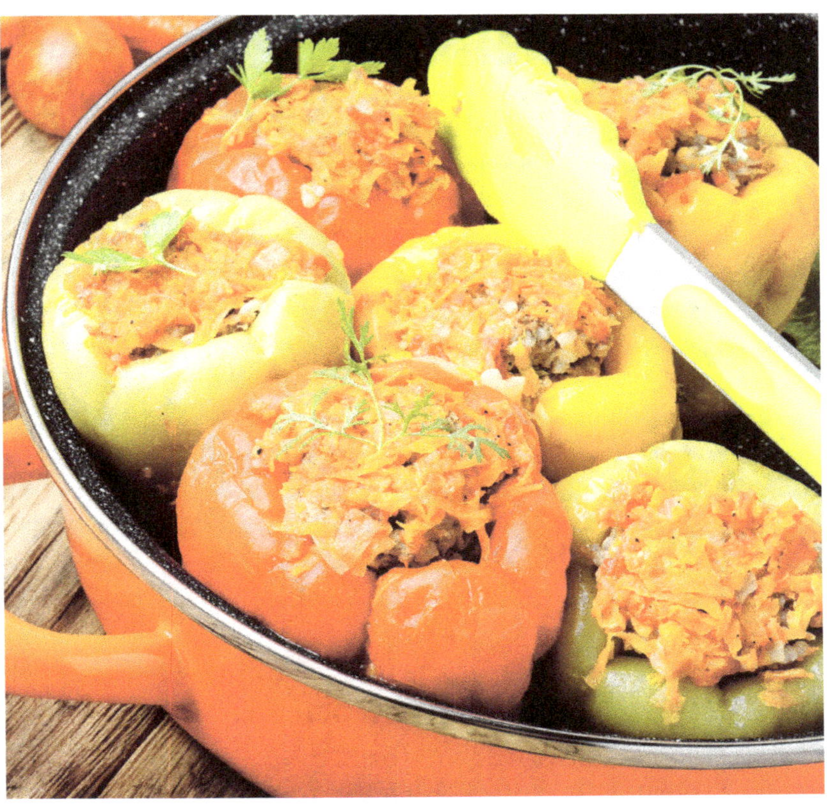

Directions

1. Adjust the oven's heat to 375°F (190°C).
2. Combine the broccoli, quinoa, and half of the cheddar cheese in a large bowl. Drizzle some oil over the dish and sprinkle salt and pepper for seasoning. Mix well.
3. Fill each bell pepper with the broccoli and quinoa, pressing down gently to pack the filling.
4. Place the stuffed peppers in a cooking dish and sprinkle the cheddar cheese.
5. To prepare, cover the dish with aluminum foil and bake for 25-30 minutes until the peppers become tender. Serve warm.

ZUCCHINI NOODLE PASTA WITH PESTO

Prep time
20 Min

Cook Time
10 Min

Servings
2

Nutrition Information

Calories: 280   Carbs: 12g
Protein: 7g   Fats: 23g

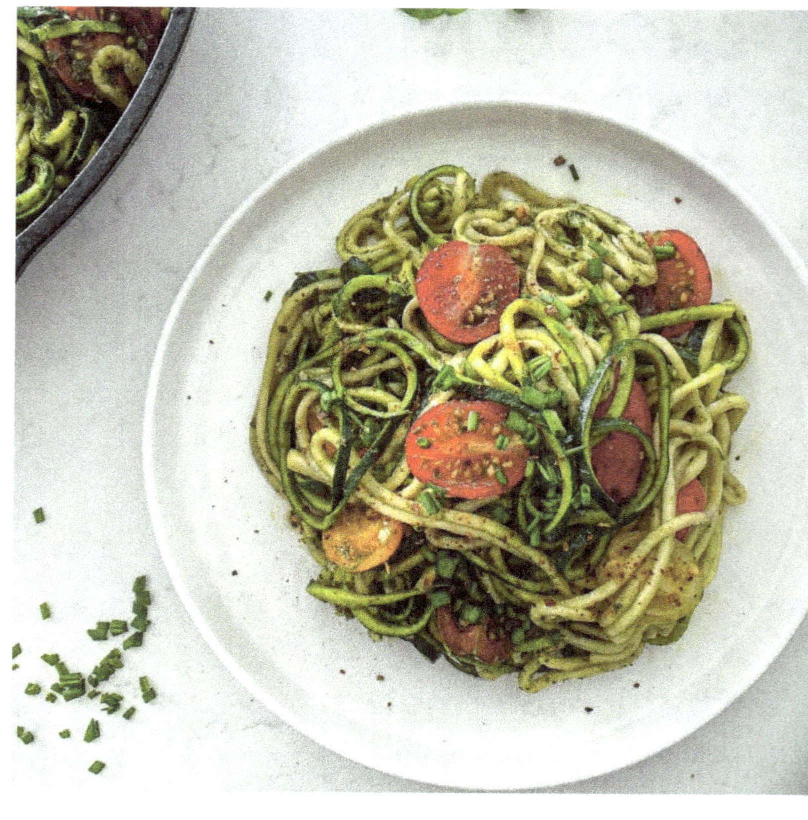

Ingredients

- 2 medium zucchinis, spiralized into noodles
- 1/2 cup basil pesto (store-bought or homemade)
- 1/4 cup cherry tomatoes, halved
- 2 tbsp grated parmesan cheese
- Salt and ground black pepper to taste

Directions

1. Warm up one tablespoon of oil over moderate heat in a large skillet. Add the zucchini noodles and sauté for 3-5 minutes until it softens slightly but still al dente.
2. Remove heat and toss the zucchini noodles with the basil pesto until well coated.
3. Divide the pasta between two plates, top with cherry tomatoes, and sprinkle with parmesan cheese.
4. Season with salt and pepper if desired. Serve immediately.

SPICED LENTIL AND CARROT SALAD

Prep time
20 Min

Cook Time
25 Min

Servings
3

Nutrition Information

Calories: 290
Protein: 13g

Carbs: 30g
Fats: 14g

Ingredients

- 1 cup dried lentils, rinsed and drained
- 2 large carrots, shredded
- 1/2 cup fresh parsley, chopped
- 1/4 cup olive oil
- 2 tsp cumin powder
- 1 lemon, juiced
- Salt and ground black pepper to taste

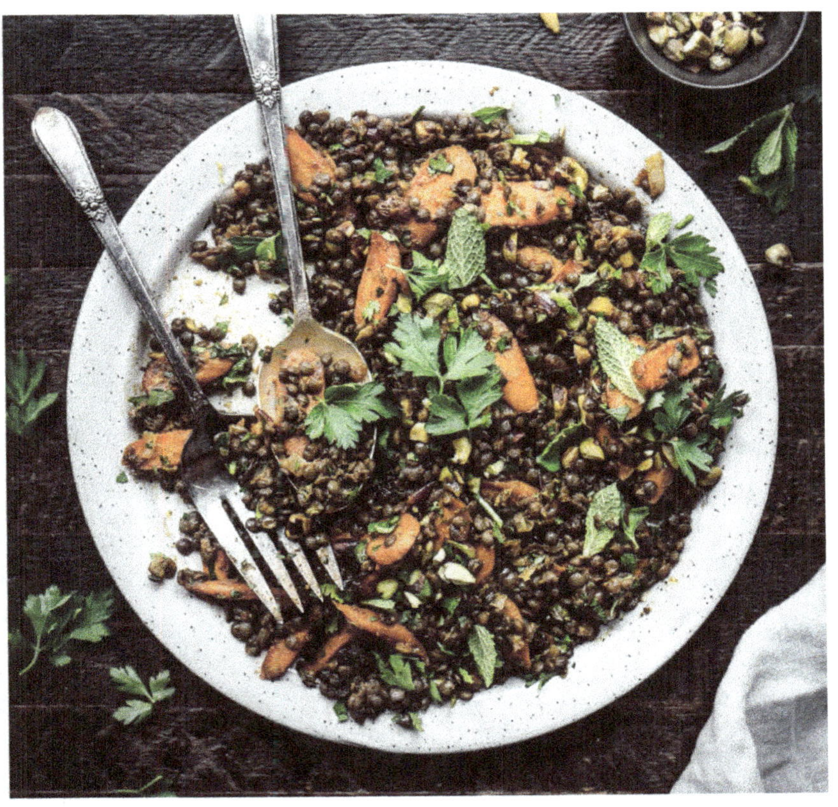

Directions

1. In a pot, get 3 cups of water to a boil. Add the lentils and cook for 20-25 minutes or until tender. Drain and set aside to cool.
2. Combine the cooked lentils, shredded carrots, and chopped parsley in a large bowl.
3. Mix the olive oil, cumin powder, and lemon juice in a small bowl—season with salt and pepper.
4. Combine the salad ingredients and then pour the dressing over them. Mix everything well. Chill for at least 30 minutes before serving.

GREEK YOGURT WITH NUTS AND HONEY

Prep time
5 Min

Cook Time
0 Min

Servings
1

Nutrition Information

Calories: 240 Carbs: 25g
Protein: 20g Fats: 7g

Ingredients

- 1 cup plain Greek yogurt
- 2 tbsp mixed nuts (like almonds, walnuts, and cashews)
- 1 tbsp honey

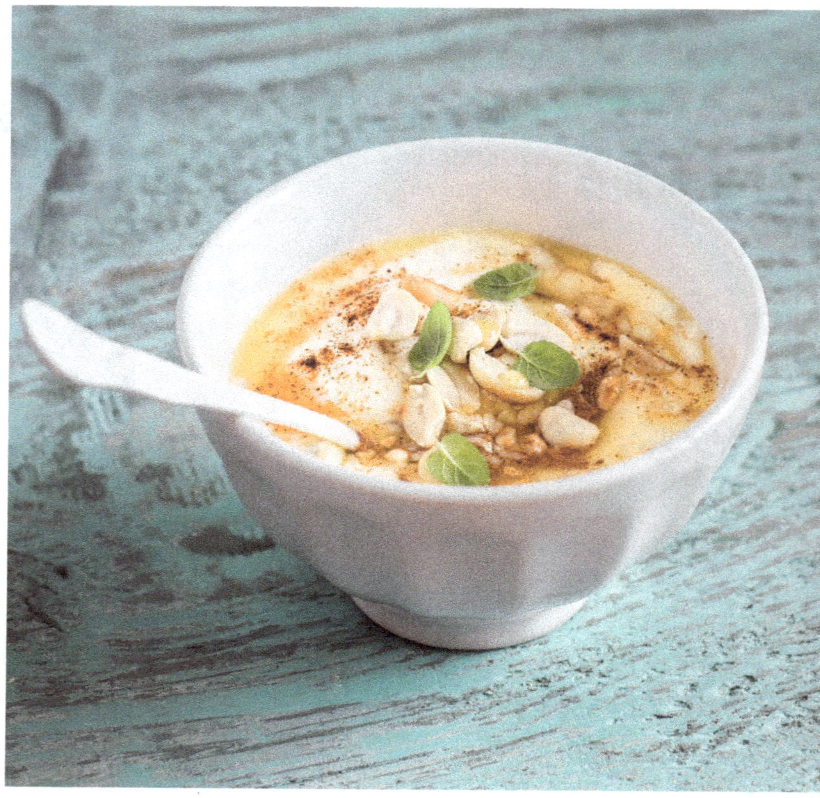

Directions

1. Spoon Greek yogurt into a serving bowl.
2. Drizzle with honey and sprinkle with mixed nuts.
3. Stir gently to combine or enjoy the layers as they are.

APPLE CINNAMON OAT BRAN MUFFINS

Prep time
20 Min

Cook Time
20 Min

Servings
6 Muffins

Nutrition Information

Calories: 160   Carbs: 35g
Protein: 5g   Fats: 2.5g

Ingredients

- 1 cup oat bran
- 1/2 cup whole wheat flour
- 1 large apple, grated
- 1/4 cup honey
- 1 tsp baking powder
- 1 tsp cinnamon powder
- 2/3 cup almond milk
- 1 egg

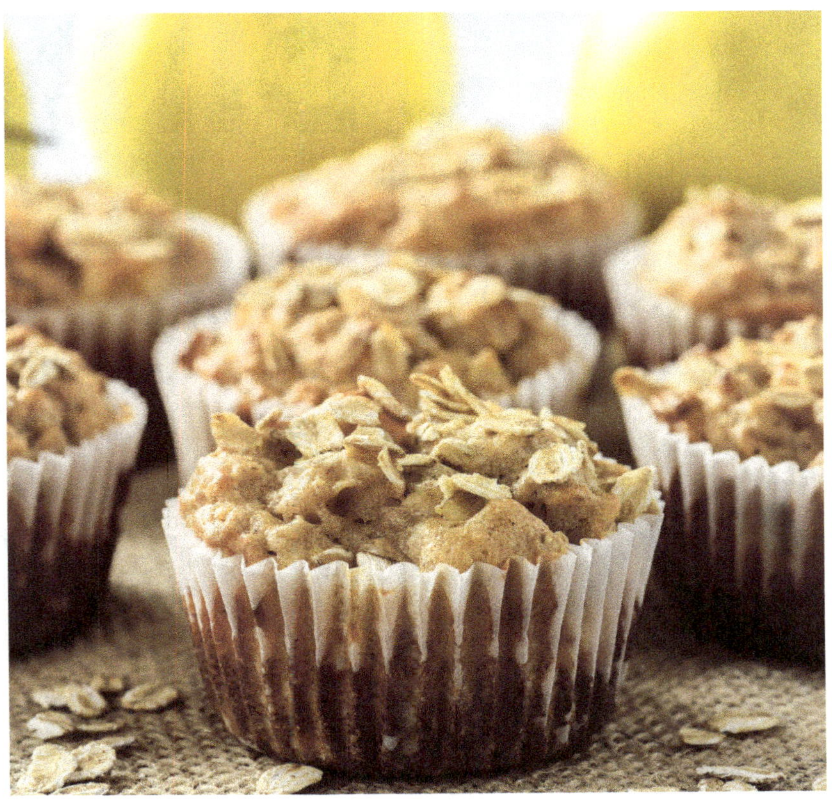

Directions

1. Set the oven's heat to 375°F (190°C) and place a muffin tin with paper liners.
2. Combine oat bran, whole wheat flour, baking powder, and cinnamon in a large bowl.
3. Whisk together the almond milk, egg, and honey in another bowl. Stir in the grated apple.
4. Combine the wet & dry ingredients only until they are mixed. Then, evenly pour the batter into the muffin cups and bake for approximately 18-20 minutes. Check if the muffins are cooked by entering a toothpick in the center. If it comes out clean, then the muffins are done. Cool on a wire rack.

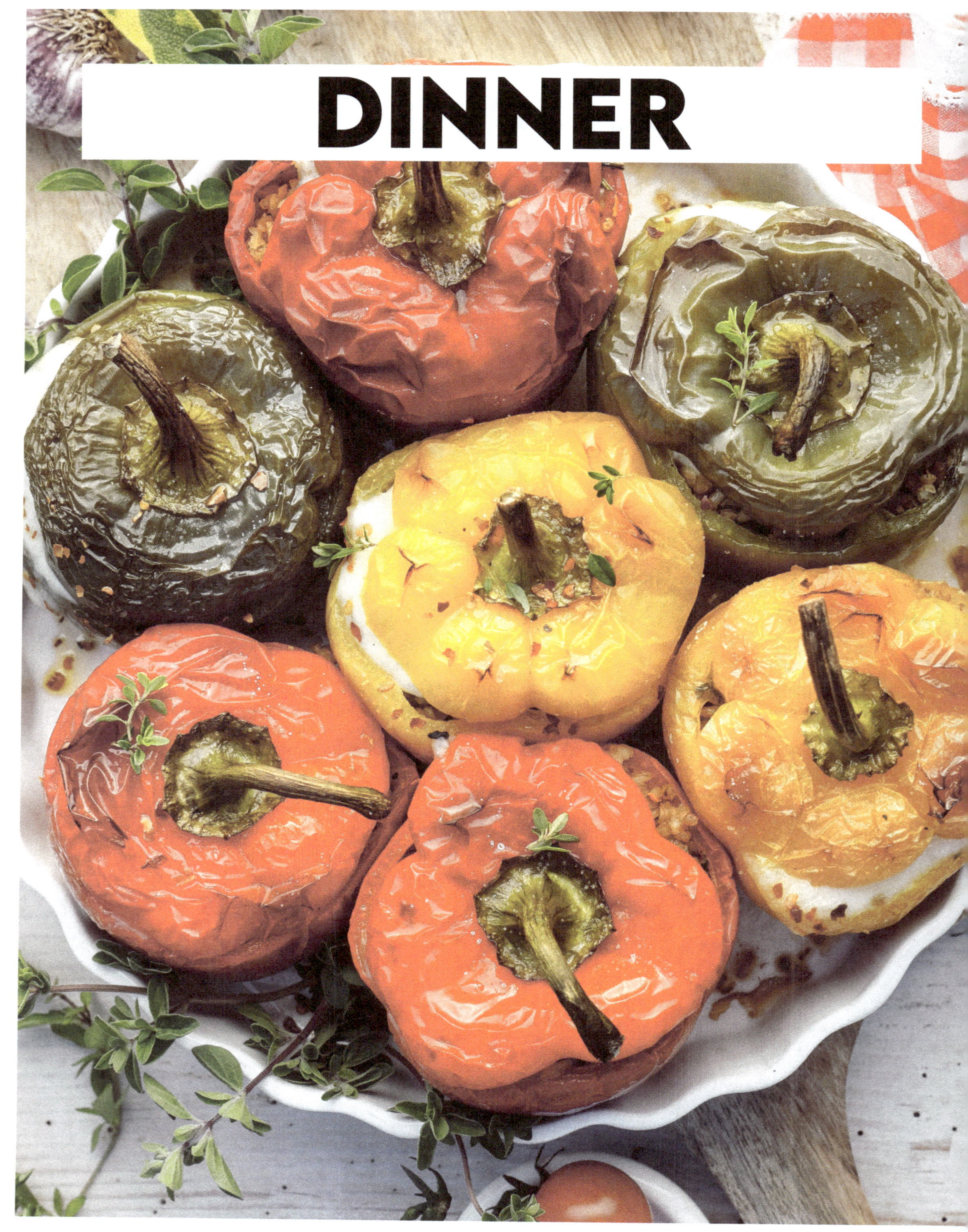

DINNER

GRILLED EGGPLANT AND SPINACH SALAD

Prep time
15 Min

Cook Time
10 Min

Servings
2

Nutrition Information

Calories: 210   Carbs: 18g
Protein: 6g   Fats: 14g

Ingredients

- 1 large eggplant, sliced
- 2 cups fresh spinach
- 1/4 cup feta cheese, crumbled
- 2 tbsp olive oil
- 1 lemon, juiced
- Salt and ground black pepper to taste

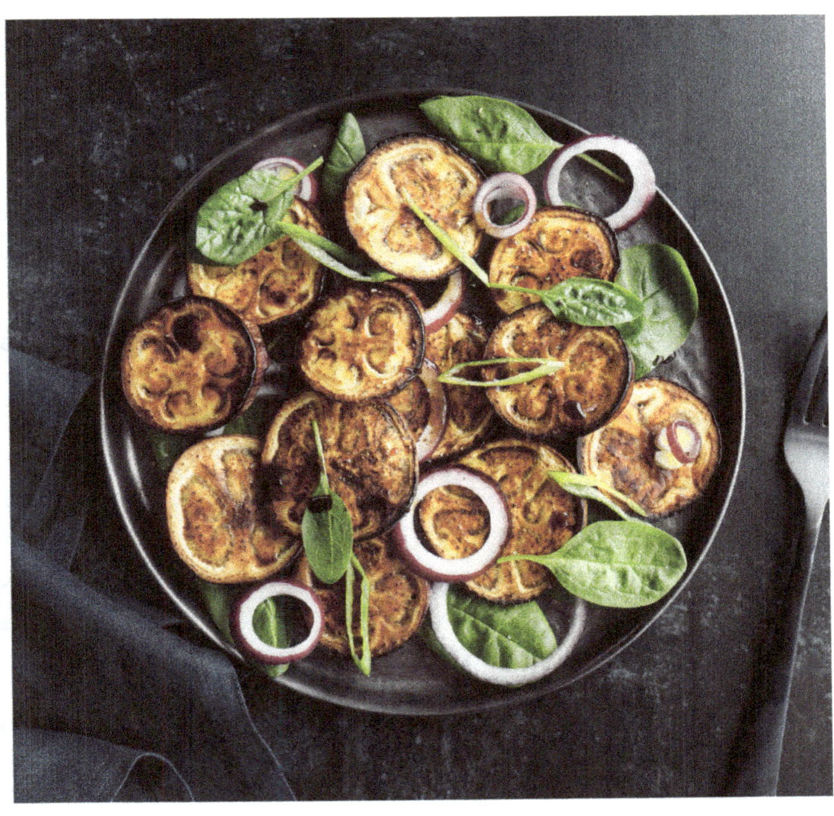

Directions

1. Preheat the grill or grill pan over medium heat.
2. First, apply a layer of olive oil to the eggplant slices. Then, sprinkle some salt and pepper to enhance the flavor.
3. Grill the eggplant slices on each side for 4-5 minutes until charred and soft.
4. Arrange the spinach on plates, top with grilled eggplant slices, crumbled feta cheese, and drizzle with lemon juice. Serve immediately.

LEMON GARLIC ROASTED CHICKEN

Prep time
10 Min

Cook Time
45 Min

Servings
4

Nutrition Information

Calories: 280   Carbs: 5g
Protein: 28g   Fats: 16g

Ingredients

- 4 chicken breasts, boneless and skinless
- 4 garlic cloves, minced
- 2 lemons, zested and juiced
- 2 tbsp olive oil
- Fresh herbs (like rosemary and thyme)
- Salt and ground black pepper to taste

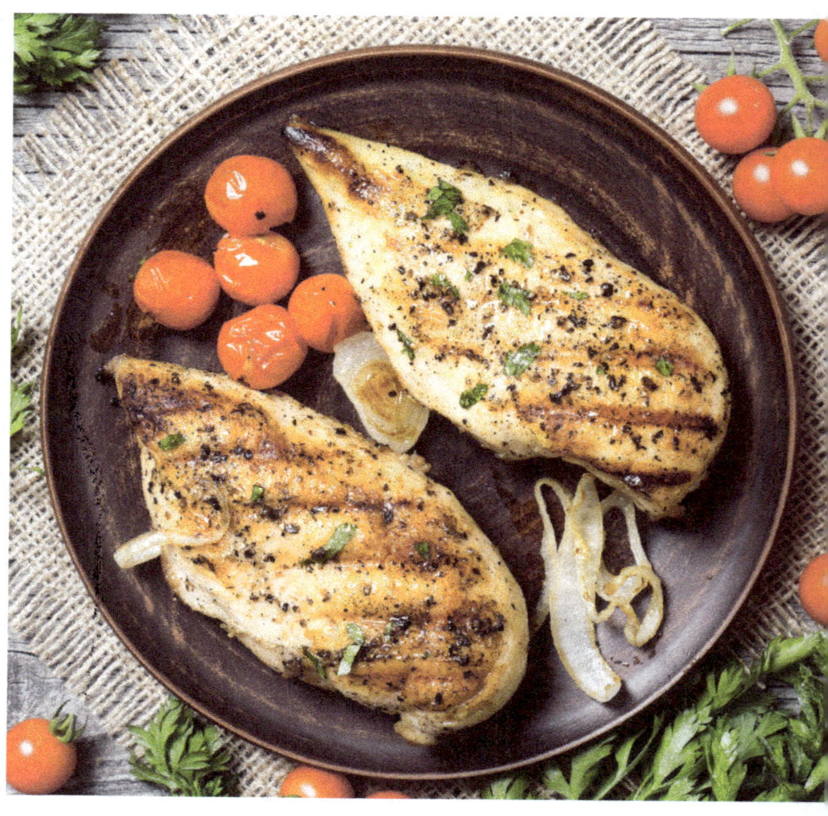

Directions

1. Set the oven's heat to 375°F (190°C).
2. Combine olive oil, lemon zest, lemon juice, garlic, and herbs in a bowl.
3. Rub the chicken breasts with the blending and season generously using salt and pepper.
4. To cook the chicken, put it in a roasting pan and bake it for 40-45 minutes or until thoroughly cooked. Baste occasionally with its juices. You can pair this dish with steamed vegetables or a salad for a complete meal.

VEGETABLE STIR-FRY WITH TOFU

Prep time
20 Min

Cook Time
15 Min

Servings
3

Nutrition Information

Calories: 250   Carbs: 20g
Protein: 15g   Fats: 12g

Ingredients

- 1 block of firm tofu, cubed
- 2 cups mixed vegetables (broccoli, bell peppers, snap peas, carrots)
- 2 tbsp soy sauce (low sodium)
- 1 tbsp sesame oil
- 1 tsp ginger, grated
- 1 garlic clove, minced
- Crushed red pepper flakes (optional)

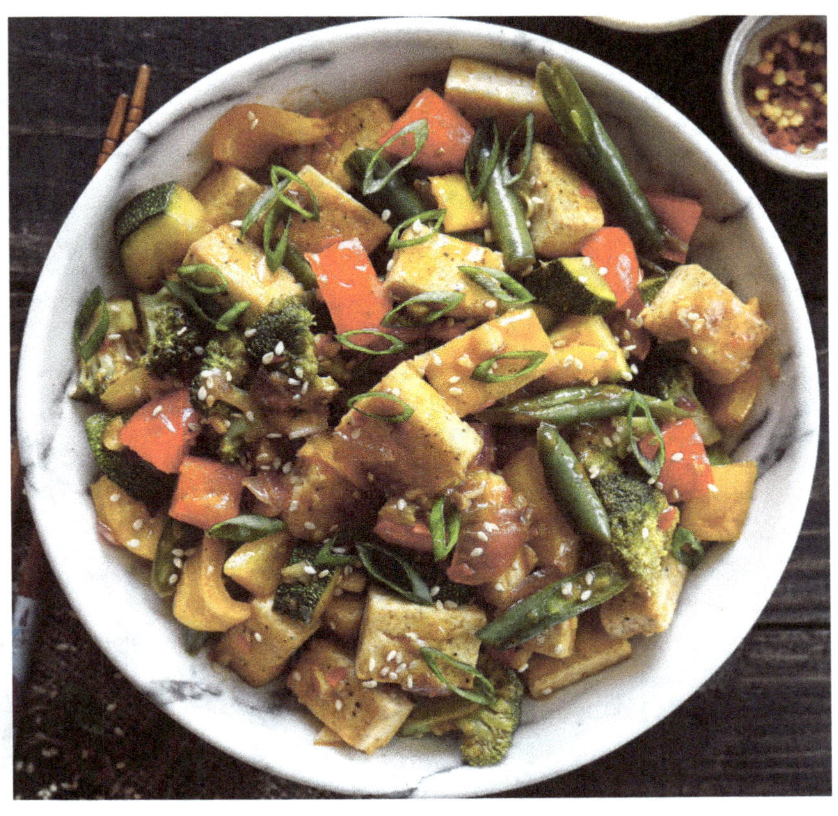

Directions

1. Heat sesame oil in a large-sized skillet or wok over medium-high heat. Add garlic and ginger, and sauté for 1 minute.
2. Add tofu cubes and cook until it gets golden brown on all sides.
3. Add the mixed vegetables and stir-fry for 7-10 minutes or until veggies are tender-crisp.
4. Drizzle with soy sauce and sprinkle with red pepper flakes if desired. Serve hot with brown rice or quinoa.

SPAGHETTI SQUASH WITH TOMATO BASIL SAUCE

Prep time
10 Min

Cook Time
45 Min

Servings
4

Nutrition Information

Calories: 160   Carbs: 30g
Protein: 3g   Fats: 5g

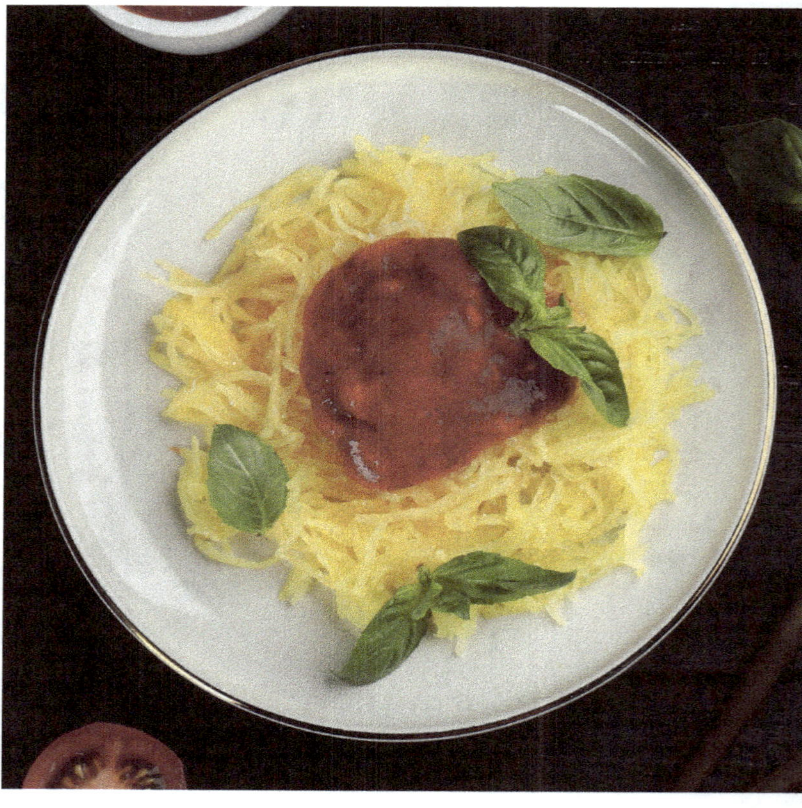

Ingredients

- 1 large spaghetti squash
- 2 cups tomato sauce (homemade or low sodium store-bought)
- 2 garlic cloves, minced
- Fresh basil leaves
- 1 tbsp olive oil
- Salt and ground black pepper to taste
- Grated parmesan cheese (optional)

Directions

1. Set the oven's heat to 400°F (200°C) to cook spaghetti squash. To prepare the squash, cut it in half lengthwise and then remove the seeds.
2. Place the squash cut-side on a baking sheet and bake for 40-45 minutes, or until the flesh quickly shreds with a fork.
3. In a saucepan, warm olive oil over moderate heat. Add garlic and sauté until fragrant. To the mixture, incorporate tomato sauce and season it with salt and pepper. Then, allow it to simmer for ten minutes.
4. Once the squash is prepared, scrape the "spaghetti" strands with a fork. Serve with tomato sauce, fresh basil leaves, and optional parmesan cheese.

BALSAMIC GLAZED SALMON

Prep time
15 Min

Cook Time
20 Min

Servings
4

Nutrition Information

Calories: 310   Carbs: 12g
Protein: 25g   Fats: 18g

Ingredients

- 4 salmon fillets
- 1/4 cup balsamic vinegar
- 2 tbsp honey
- 2 garlic cloves, minced
- Salt and ground black pepper to taste
- Fresh dill for garnish

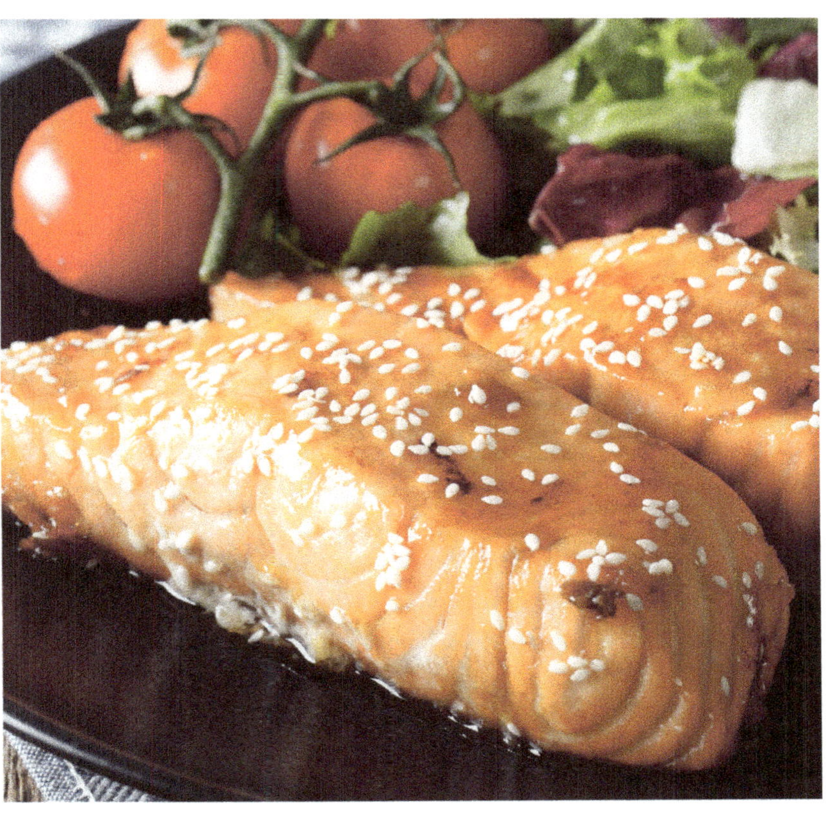

Directions

1. Set the oven's heat to 400°F (200°C).
2. In a small-sized saucepan, combine balsamic vinegar, honey, and garlic. Let it simmer for 5-7 minutes until it thickens a bit.
3. To prepare the salmon fillets, sprinkle salt and pepper on both sides. Then, place them on a baking tray.
4. Brush the balsamic glaze over the salmon.
5. Prepare for 15-20 minutes or until salmon flakes easily with a fork.
6. Garnish with fresh dill before serving.

LENTIL AND MUSHROOM STUFFED BELL PEPPERS

Prep time
20 Min

Cook Time
30 Min

Servings
4

Nutrition Information

Calories: 220
Protein: 10g

Carbs: 30g
Fats: 7g

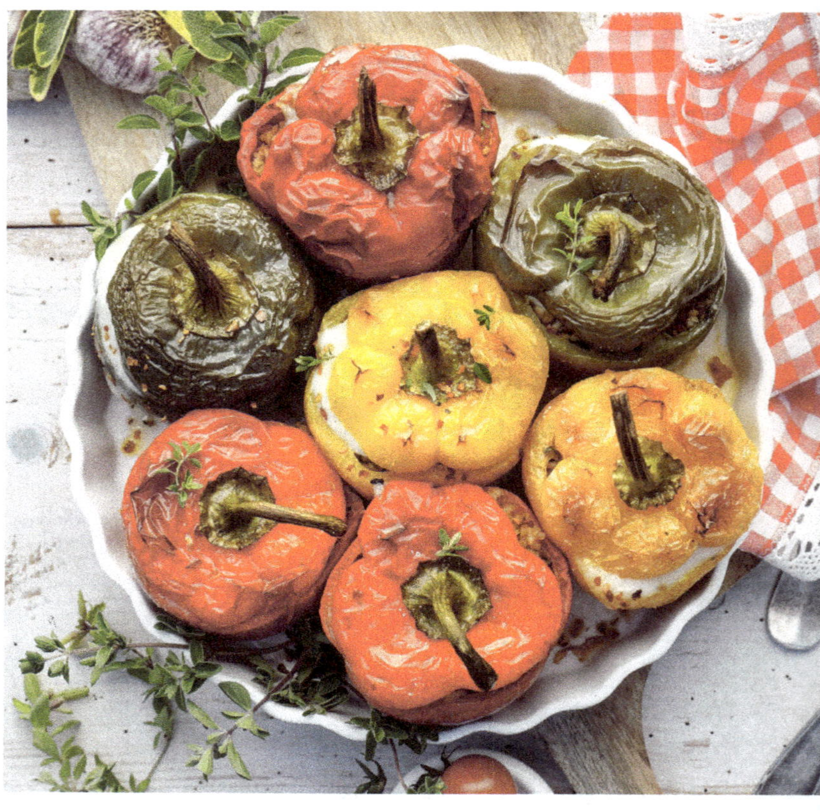

Ingredients

- 4 bell peppers (any color)
- 1 cup cooked lentils
- 1 cup mushrooms, chopped
- 1 onion, chopped
- 2 garlic cloves, minced
- 1 tbsp olive oil
- Salt and ground black pepper to taste
- Fresh parsley, chopped (for garnish)

Directions

1. Adjust the oven's temperature to 375°F (190°C).
2. In a pan, heat olive oil and sauté onions and garlic until translucent.
3. Add mushrooms and prepare for another 5 minutes.
4. Add the prepared lentils to the mixture and season it with salt and pepper.
5. To prepare bell peppers, cut off their tops and remove the seeds. Fill each pepper with the lentil and mushroom mixture.
6. Place the stuffed peppers in a cooking dish and cover with foil.
7. Bake for 25-30 minutes. Garnish with fresh parsley before serving.

GINGER STIR-FRIED SHRIMP WITH BROCCOLI

Prep time
15 Min

Cook Time
15 Min

Servings
4

Nutrition Information

Calories: 250   Carbs: 10g
Protein: 25g   Fats: 12g

Ingredients

- 1 lb shrimp, peeled and deveined
- 2 cups broccoli florets
- 1 tbsp ginger, minced
- 3 garlic cloves, minced
- 2 tbsp soy sauce (low sodium)
- 2 tbsp sesame oil
- Red pepper flakes (optional)

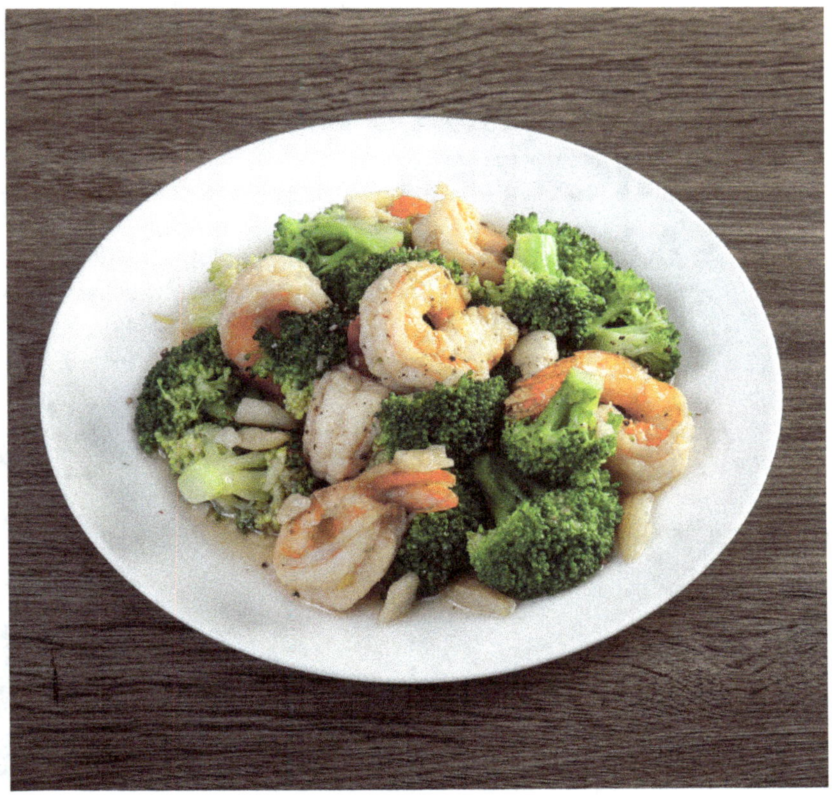

Directions

1. Heat sesame oil in a wok or large-sized skillet over medium-high heat.
2. Add ginger and garlic, stirring for a minute until fragrant.
3. Place the shrimp into the pan and cook them until they turn pink.
4. Add broccoli florets, soy sauce, and red pepper flakes (if using). Stir-fry for another 5-7 minutes until broccoli is tender.
5. Serve immediately with a s de of brown rice or quinoa.

HERB-GRILLED ZUCCHINI AND CHICKPEA SALAD

 **Prep time**
20 Min

 **Cook Time**
10 Min

 **Servings**
4

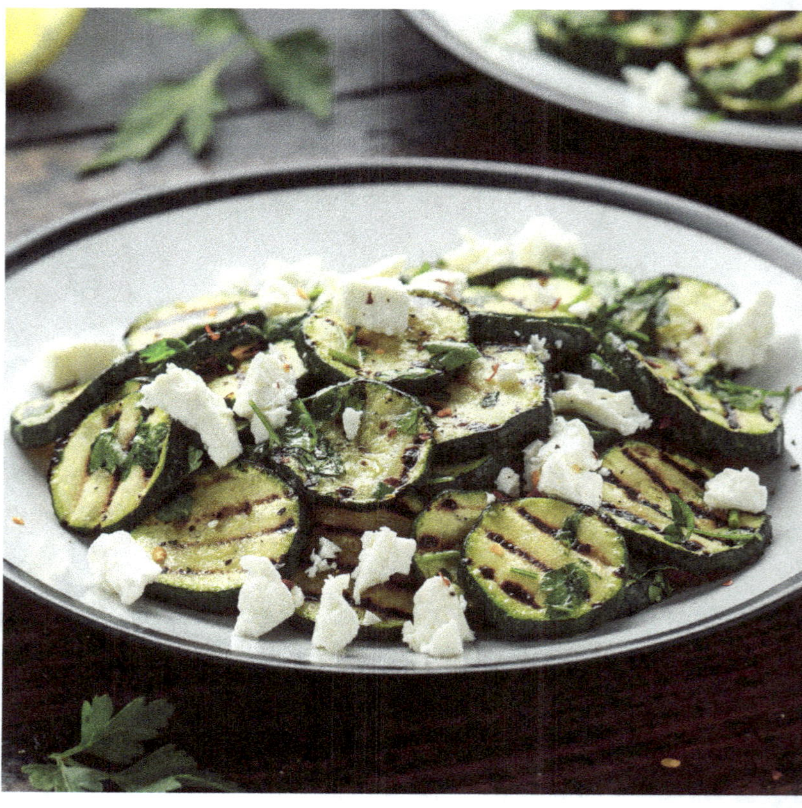

Nutrition Information

Calories: 230
Protein: 8g

Carbs: 25g
Fats: 12g

Ingredients

- 2 zucchinis, sliced lengthwise
- 1 can chickpeas, drained and rinsed
- 1/4 cup fresh mint, chopped
- 1/4 cup fresh parsley, chopped
- 2 tbsp olive oil
- Juice of 1 lemon
- Salt and ground black pepper to taste

Directions

1. Preheat the grill or grill pan over medium heat.
2. Brush zucchini slices with some olive oil and season with salt and pepper.
3. Grill zucchini on each side for 3-4 minutes until charred and soft.
4. In a large bowl, combine grilled zucchini, chickpeas, mint, parsley, olive oil, and lemon juice. Toss well.
5. Season with extra salt & pepper, if needed. Serve chilled or at room temperature.

ROASTED BUTTERNUT SQUASH AND SPINACH CURRY

Prep time
20 Min

Cook Time
35 Min

Servings
4

Nutrition Information

Calories: 290
Protein: 4g

Carbs: 32g
Fats: 18g

Ingredients

- 1 medium butternut squash, peeled and cubed
- 2 cups fresh spinach
- 1 onion, chopped
- 2 garlic cloves, minced
- 1 tbsp fresh ginger, minced
- 2 tbsp coconut oil
- 2 tbsp curry powder
- 1 can coconut milk (14 oz)
- Salt and ground black pepper to taste
- Fresh cilantro for garnish

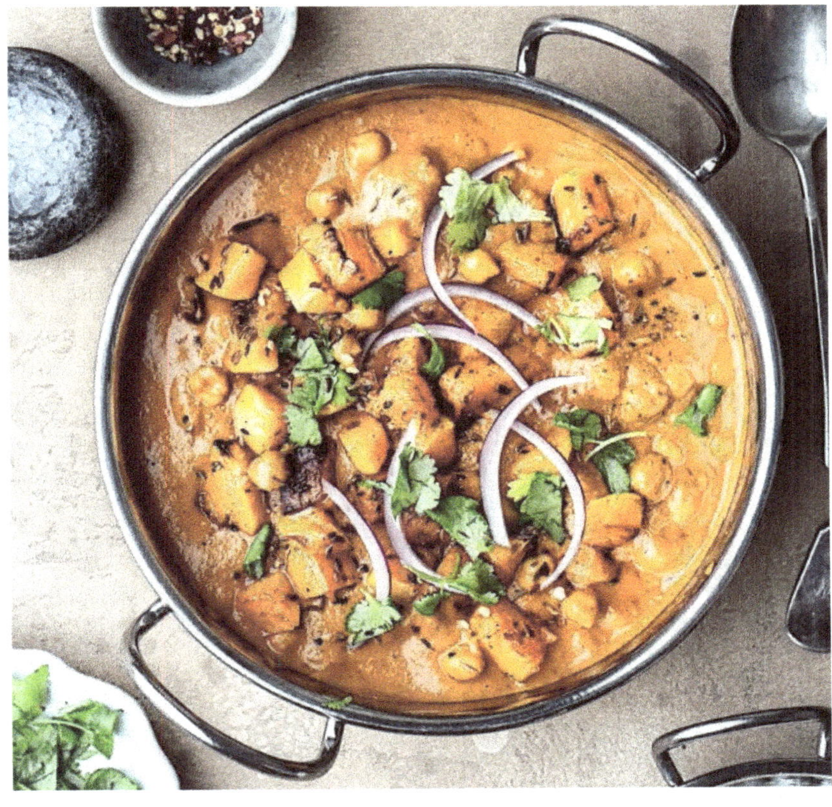

Directions

1. Set the oven's heat to 400°F (200°C) to prepare for baking.
2. Mix 1 tablespoon of coconut oil, salt, & pepper with the cubed squash to prepare the butternut squash. Spread the blending on a baking sheet and roast in the oven for 20-25 minutes or until the squash is soft and tender.
3. In a large skillet, heat the remaining coconut oil over medium heat. Add onions, garlic, and ginger, sautéing until translucent
4. After adding the curry powder, continue cooking for two more minutes.
5. Pour in the coconut milk, taking it to a gentle simmer. Add the roasted butternut squash and fresh spinach, stirring until the spinach is wilted.
6. If necessary, add more salt and pepper to the season. Serve the curry warm, garnished with fresh cilantro.

GROUND TURKEY AND GREEN BEAN STIR-FRY

Prep time
15 Min

Cook Time
20 Min

Servings
4

Nutrition Information

Calories: 240   Carbs: 10g
Protein: 22g   Fats: 12g

Ingredients

- 1 lb ground turkey
- 2 cups of green beans, cut into bite-sized pieces
- 1 onion, chopped
- 2 garlic cloves, minced
- 2 tbsp soy sauce (low sodium)
- 1 tbsp sesame oil
- 1 tbsp ground ginger
- Crushed red pepper flakes (optional)

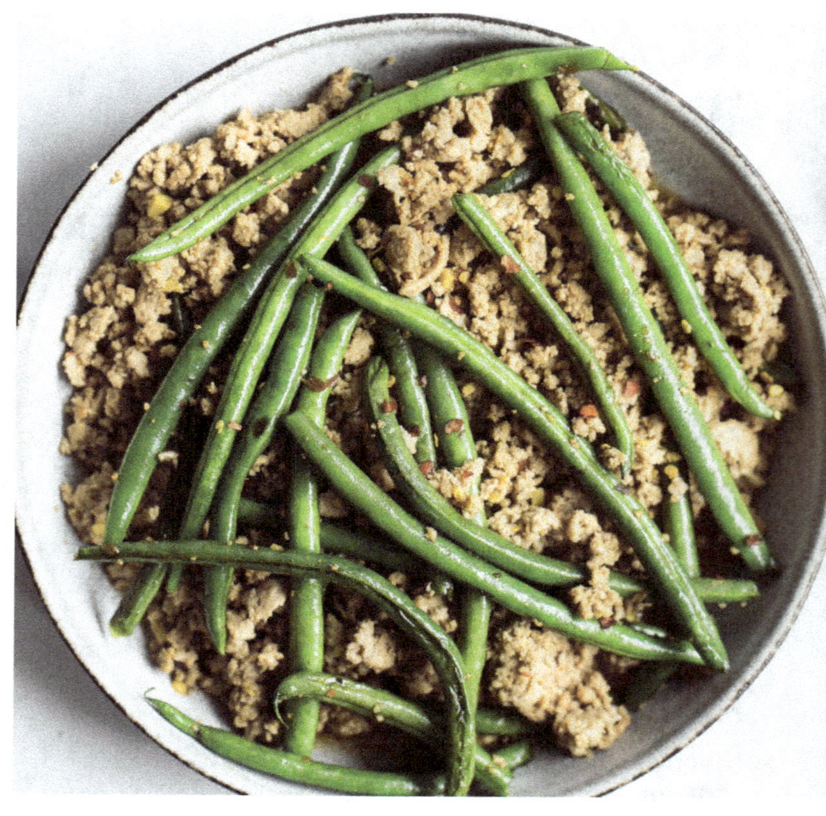

Directions

1. In a large-sized skillet or wok, heat sesame oil over medium-high heat. Add onions and garlic, stirring until translucent.
2. Add the ground turkey, cook until browned, and break it into small pieces.
3. Stir in the green beans, soy sauce, ground ginger, and red pepper flakes (if using). Cook for another 7-10 minutes until the green beans are tender-crisp.
4. To enjoy the dish, serve it hot with quinoa or brown rice.

CREAMY AVOCADO BASIL SPAGHETTI SQUASH

Prep time
20 Min

Cook Time
40 Min

Servings
4

Nutrition Information

Calories: 270

Carbs: 30g

Protein: 3g

Fats: 18g

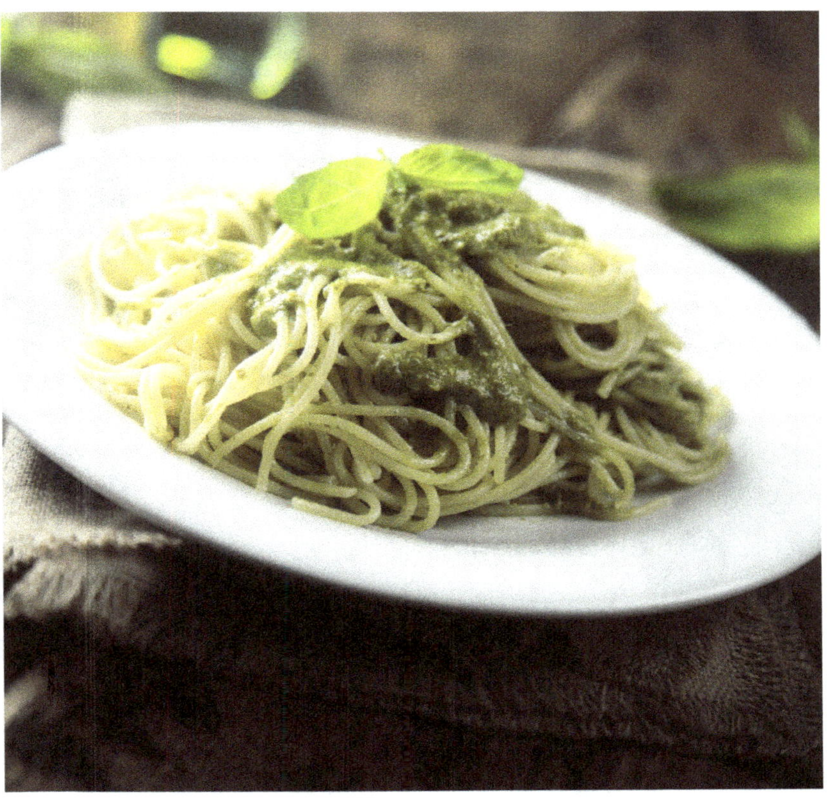

Ingredients

- 1 large spaghetti squash
- 2 ripe avocados
- 1/2 cup fresh basil
- 2 garlic cloves
- Juice of 1 lemon
- 2 tbsp olive oil
- Salt and ground black pepper to taste
- Cherry tomatoes, halved (for garnish)

Directions

1. Set the oven's heat to 400°F (200°C). Cut the spaghetti squash in half lengthwise and take out the seeds.
2. Place the halves cut side on a cooking sheet and roast for 40 minutes or until it gets tender.
3. Combine avocados, basil, garlic, lemon juice, olive oil, salt, and pepper in a blender. Blend until smooth.
4. After cooking the spaghetti squash, use a fork to scrape out its flesh and create strands that resemble spaghetti.
5. Toss the squash with the creamy avocado basil sauce. Garnish with halved cherry tomatoes before serving.

HERB ROASTED CHICKEN THIGHS WITH ASPARAGUS

 **Prep time**
10 Min

 **Cook Time**
35 Min

 **Servings**
4

Nutrition Information

Calories: 310   Carbs: 5g
Protein: 24g   Fats: 22g

Ingredients

- 4 bone-in, skin-on chicken thighs
- 1 bunch of asparagus, trimmed
- 2 tbsp olive oil
- 1 tbsp chopped fresh rosemary
- 1 tbsp chopped fresh thyme
- 2 garlic cloves, minced
- Salt and ground black pepper to taste
- Lemon wedges for serving

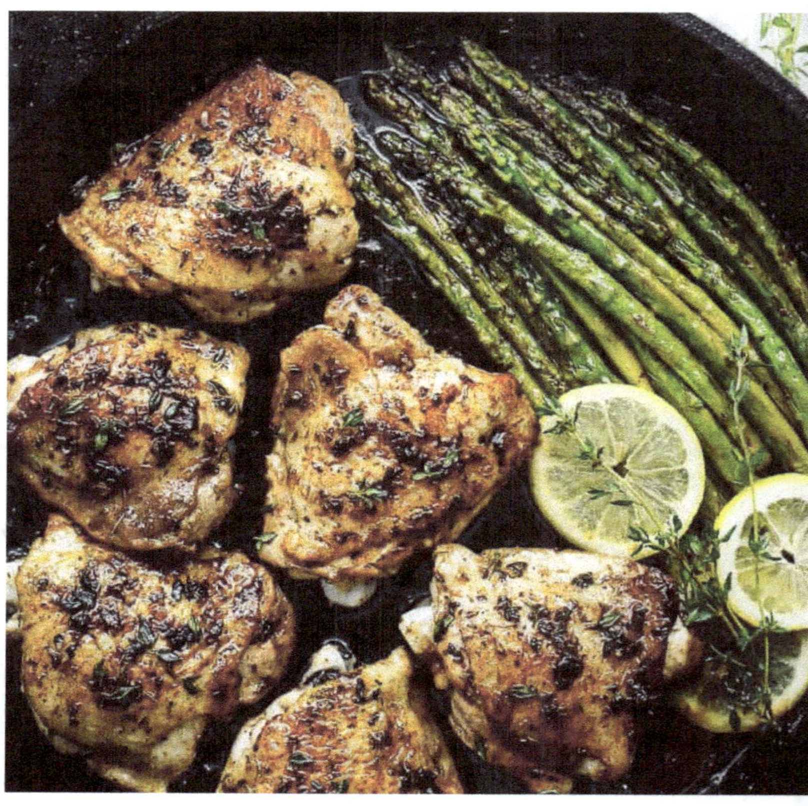

Directions

1. Set the oven's temperature to 425°F (220°C).
2. In a large-sized bowl, combine olive oil, rosemary, thyme, garlic, salt, and pepper. Add the chicken thighs and coat them thoroughly with the herb mixture.
3. Place chicken thighs on a baking tray, skin-side up. Roast for 25 minutes.
4. Remove the tray from the oven, add asparagus around the chicken thighs, and drizzle them with olive oil. Return to the oven and roast for 10-15 minutes or until chicken is golden and fully cooked and asparagus is tender.
5. Serve with lemon wedges on the side.

EGGPLANT AND CHICKPEA CURRY

Prep time
15 Min

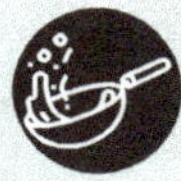

Cook Time
25 Min

Servings
4

Nutrition Information

Calories: 300
Protein: 9g
Carbs: 32g
Fats: 17g

Ingredients

- 1 large eggplant, cubed
- 1 can chickpeas, drained and rinsed
- 1 onion, chopped
- 2 tomatoes, diced
- 2 garlic cloves, minced
- 2 tbsp curry powder
- 1 can coconut milk (14 oz)
- 2 tbsp coconut oil
- Fresh cilantro, chopped (for garnish)

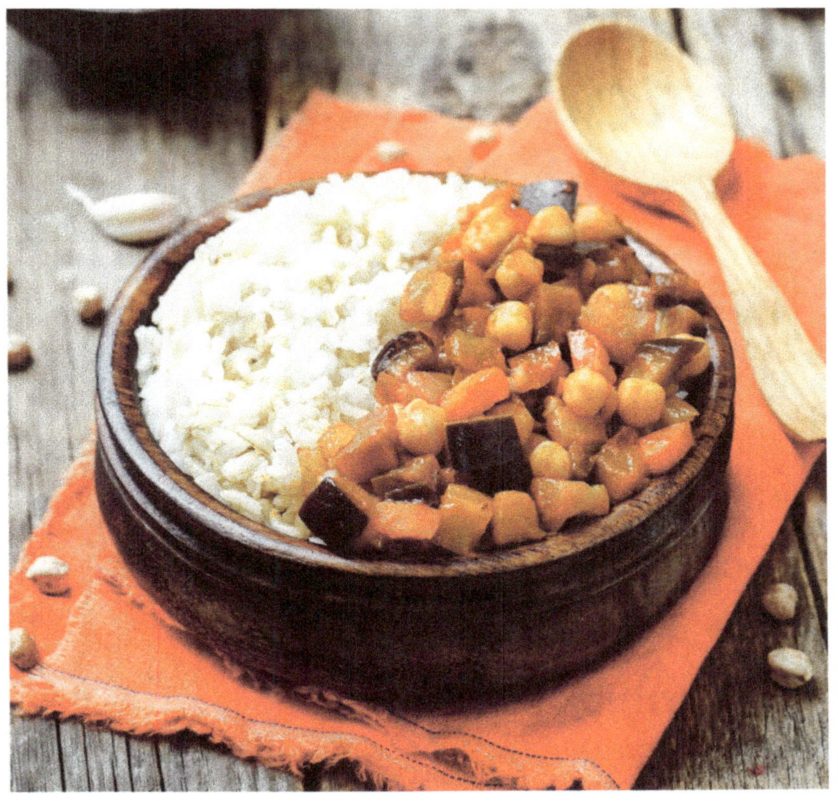

Directions

1. In a large pot or pan, heat coconut oil over medium heat. Add onions and garlic, and sauté until translucent.
2. Stir in the curry powder, cooking for about a minute until fragrant.
3. Add the diced tomatoes, eggplant cubes, and chickpeas to the pot. Mix well.
4. Pour in the coconut milk and stir. Take the mixture to a gentle simmer, then reduce the heat and let it cook for 20-25 minutes or until the eggplant is soft.
5. Garnish with fresh cilantro before serving.

BEEF AND BROCCOLI STIR-FRY

Prep time
20 Min

Cook Time
20 Min

Servings
4

Nutrition Information

Calories: 330   Carbs: 18g
Protein: 26g   Fats: 18g

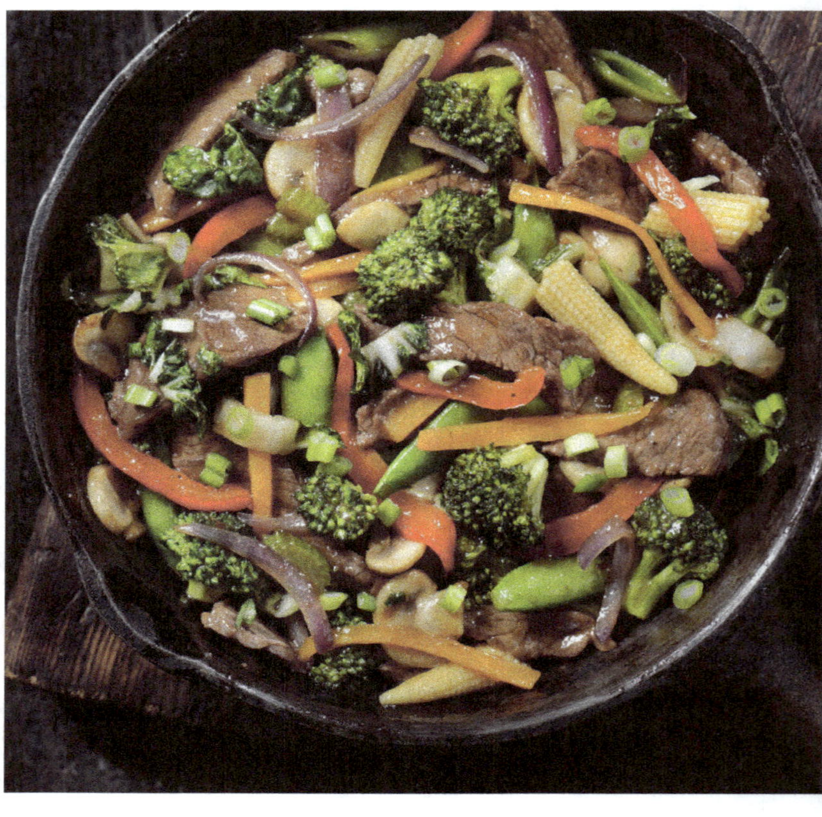

Ingredients

- 1 lb beef sirloin, thinly sliced
- 2 cups broccoli florets
- 1 bell pepper, sliced
- 3 tbsp soy sauce (low sodium)
- 1 tbsp honey
- 1 tbsp ginger, minced
- 2 garlic cloves, minced
- 1 tbsp sesame oil
- 1 tbsp olive oil

Directions

1. Mix soy sauce, honey, ginger, and garlic in a small bowl.
2. Warm oil in a large-sized skillet over medium-high heat. Add the beef slices and prepare until browned on all sides.
3. Push the beef to the side of the skillet, add sesame oil, and toss in the broccoli florets and bell pepper slices.
4. After cooking the beef and veggies, pour the soy sauce mixture on top. Stir-fry everything together for 5-7 minutes until the vegetables get tender and the meat is cooked.
5. Serve hot.

QUINOA AND ROASTED VEGGIE BOWL

Prep time
15 Min

Cook Time
25 Min

Servings
4

Nutrition Information

Calories: 270   Carbs: 42g
Protein: 7g   Fats: 8g

Ingredients

- 1 cup quinoa (cooked following package instructions)
- 1 zucchini, sliced
- 1 bell pepper, chopped
- 1 red onion, chopped
- 2 tbsp olive oil
- 2 tbsp balsamic vinegar
- Salt and ground black pepper to taste
- Feta cheese crumbles (optional)
- Fresh parsley, chopped (for garnish)

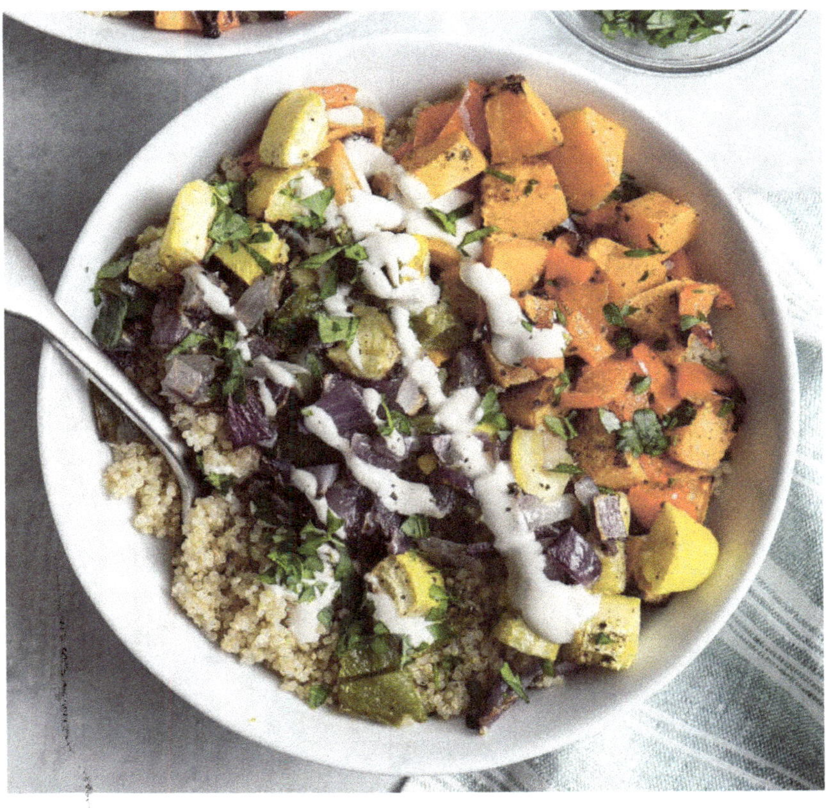

Directions

1. Set the oven's heat to 400°F (200°C).
2. Mix the zucchini, bell pepper, red onion with olive oil, balsamic vinegar, salt, and pepper. Spread them out on a baking sheet.
3. Roast the veggies for 20-25 minutes until tender and slightly caramelized.
4. In individual bowls, layer the cooked quinoa, roasted veggies, and sprinkle with feta cheese (if using). Garnish with fresh parsley.

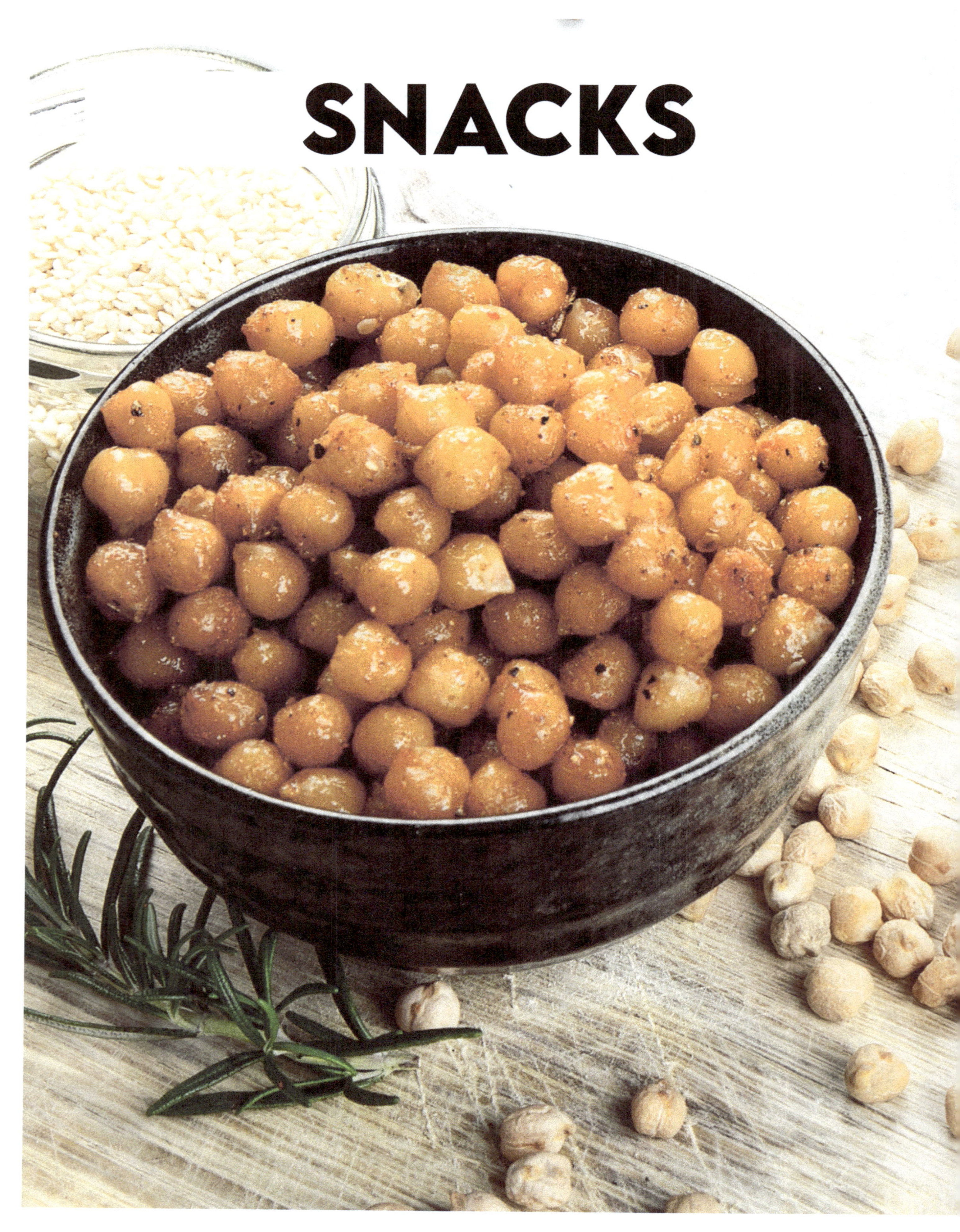
SNACKS

CUCUMBER AND HUMMUS BITES

 **Prep time**
10 Min

 **Cook Time**
0 Min

 **Servings**
4

Nutrition Information

Calories: 60   Carbs: 7g
Protein: 2g   Fats: 3g

Ingredients

- 1 large cucumber, sliced into rounds
- 1 cup hummus
- Fresh dill for garnish

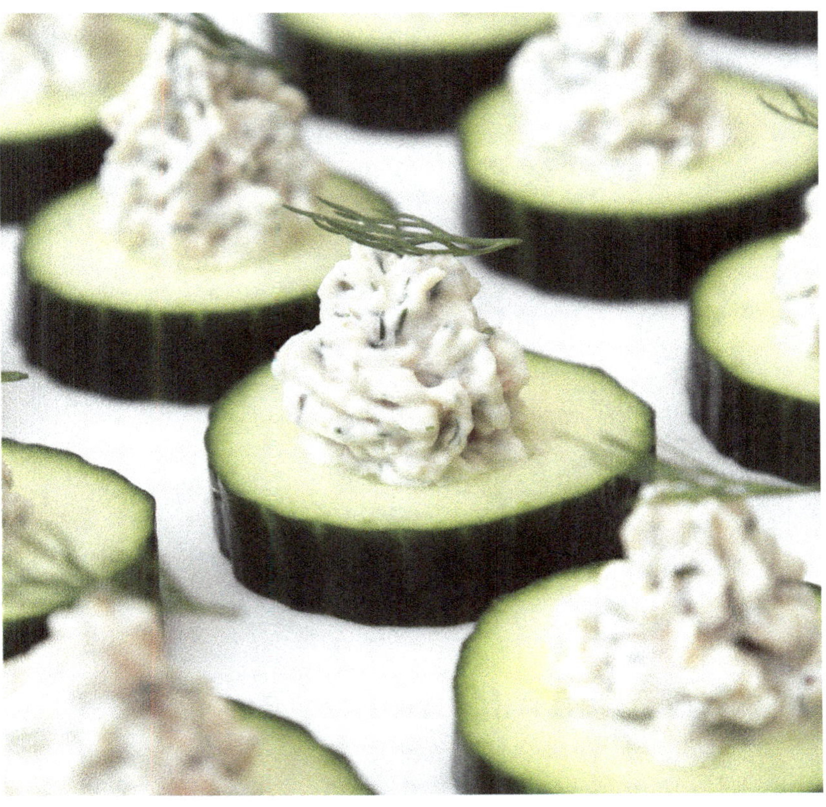

Directions

1. Lay cucumber slices flat on a serving platter.
2. Dollop a teaspoon of hummus on each piece.
3. Garnish with a sprig of fresh dill.

SPICED ROASTED CHICKPEAS

Prep time
5 Min

Cook Time
30 Min

Servings
4

Nutrition Information

Calories: 150

Carbs: 20g

Protein: 6g

Fats: 6g

Ingredients

- 1 can chickpeas, drained and rinsed
- 2 tbsp olive oil
- 1 tsp smoked paprika
- 1 tsp cumin
- Salt and ground black pepper to taste

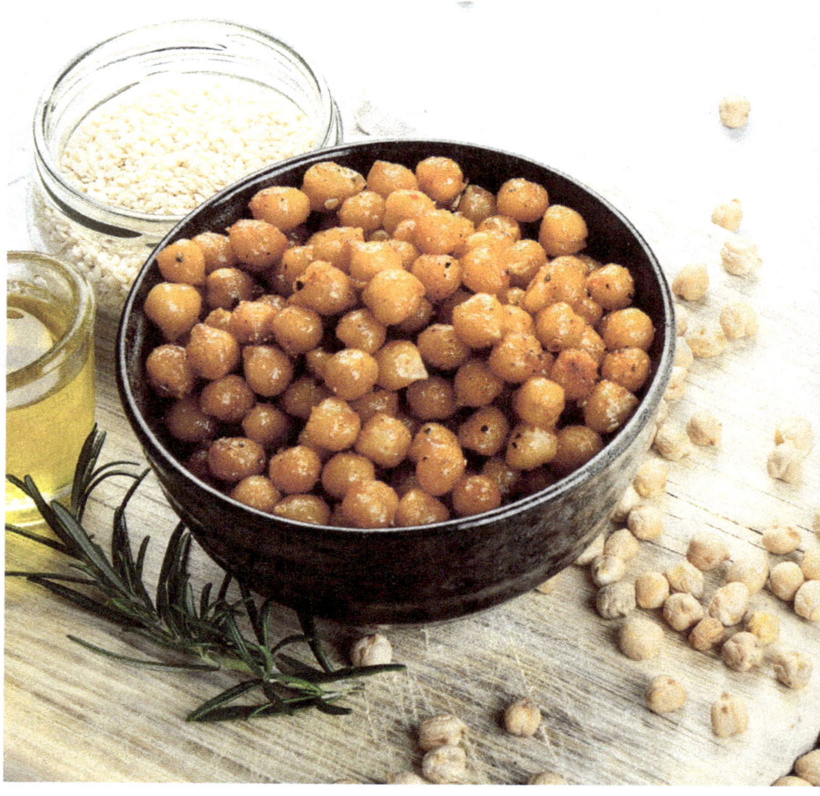

Directions

1. Preheat oven to 400°F (200°C).
2. Toss chickpeas with olive oil, paprika, cumin, salt, and pepper in a bowl.
3. Spread the ingredients on a cooking sheet in a single layer.
4. Roast for 30 minutes or until crispy, stirring halfway.

AVOCADO AND TOMATO SALSA

Prep time
10 Min

Cook Time
0 Min

Servings
4

Nutrition Information

Calories: 180   Carbs: 12g
Protein: 2g   Fats: 15g

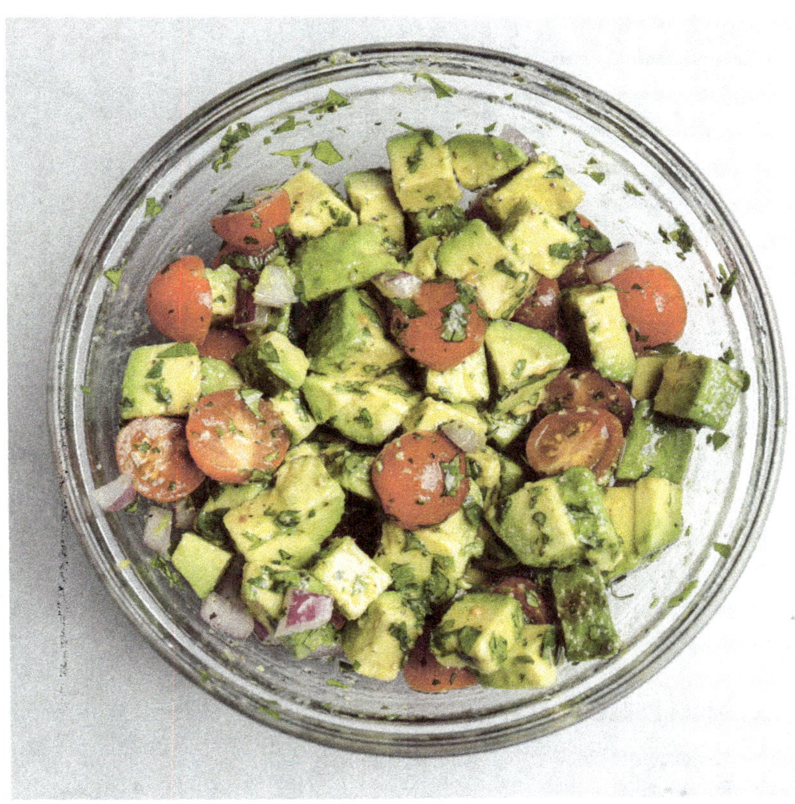

Ingredients

- 2 ripe avocados, diced
- 2 tomatoes, diced
- 1/4 onion, finely chopped
- Juice of 1 lime
- Salt and ground black pepper to taste
- Fresh cilantro, chopped

Directions

1. In a mixing bowl, combine avocados, tomatoes, and onion.
2. Drizzle with lime juice, season with salt and pepper, and toss gently.
3. Garnish with fresh cilantro.
4. Serve with whole-grain tortilla chips or vegetable sticks.

NUT AND SEED CRUNCH BARS

Prep time
15 Min

Cook Time
20 Min

Servings
8 Bars

Nutrition Information

Calories: 210   Carbs: 16g
Protein: 6g   Fats: 15g

Ingredients

- 1/2 cup almonds
- 1/2 cup cashews
- 1/4 cup pumpkin seeds
- 1/4 cup sunflower seeds
- 1/4 cup honey
- 1/4 cup almond butter

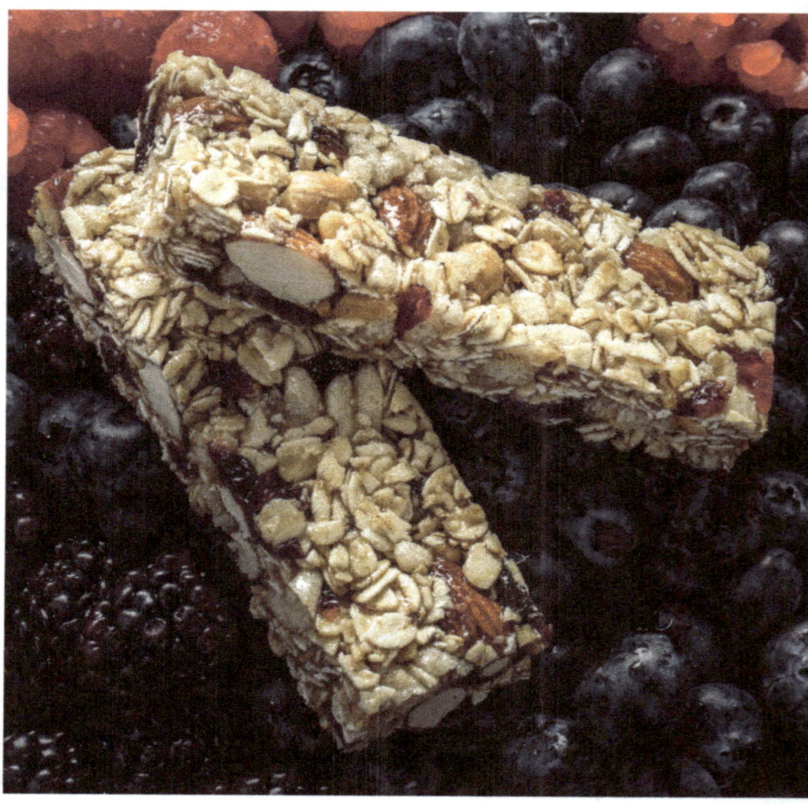

Directions

1. Preheat oven to 350°F (175°C).
2. Roughly chop almonds and cashews, and mix with pumpkin and sunflower seeds in a large-size bowl.
3. Combine honey and almond butter in another bowl until they are blended smoothly.
4. Combine wet and dry mixtures.
5. Press the blend into a square baking pan lined with parchment paper.
6. Bake for 20 minutes or until golden brown.
7. Allow to cool before cutting into bars.

BERRY ALMOND PROTEIN BITES

Prep time
15 Min

Cook Time
0 Min

Servings
12 Bites

Nutrition Information

Calories: 100   Carbs: 10g
Protein: 4g   Fats: 6g

Ingredients

- 1 cup raw almonds
- 1/2 cup dried berries (like cranberries or blueberries)
- 1/4 cup honey
- 1 scoop protein powder (preferably plant-based)
- A pinch of salt

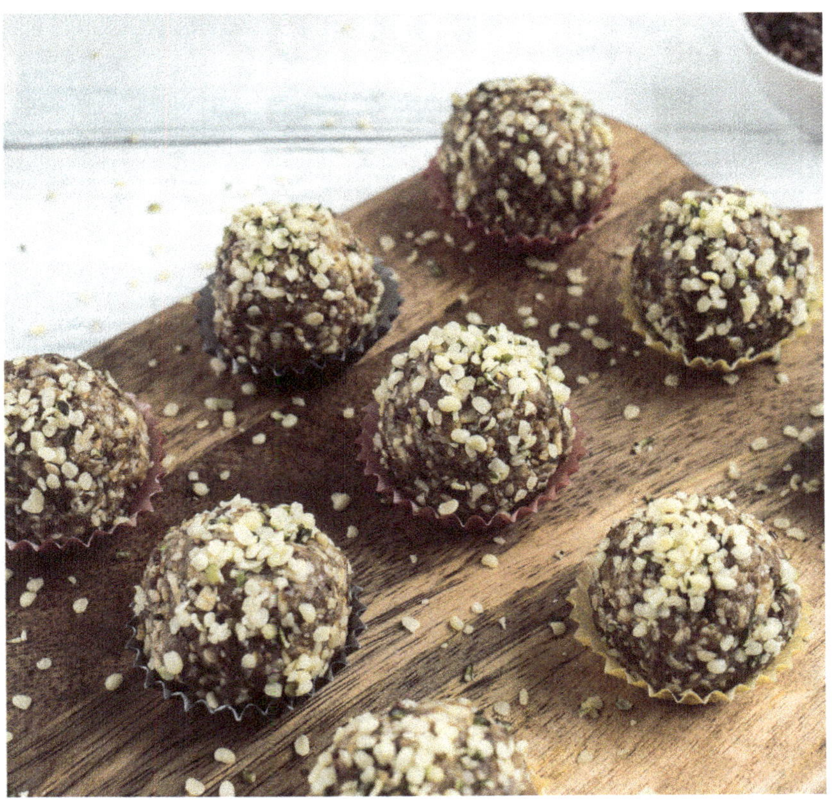

Directions

1. Using a food processor, blend almonds until they form a fine meal.
2. Add dried berries, honey, protein powder, and salt. Process until the mixture comes together.
3. Shape the blending into small balls using your hands.
4. Refrigerate for at least an hour before serving.

SPINACH AND FETA STUFFED MUSHROOMS

Prep time
15 Min

Cook Time
20 Min

Servings
4

Nutrition Information

Calories: 90   Carbs: 4g
Protein: 4g   Fats: 7g

Ingredients

- 12 large button mushrooms
- 1 cup fresh spinach, chopped
- 1/2 cup feta cheese, crumbled
- 1 garlic clove, minced
- 1 tbsp olive oil
- Salt and pepper to taste

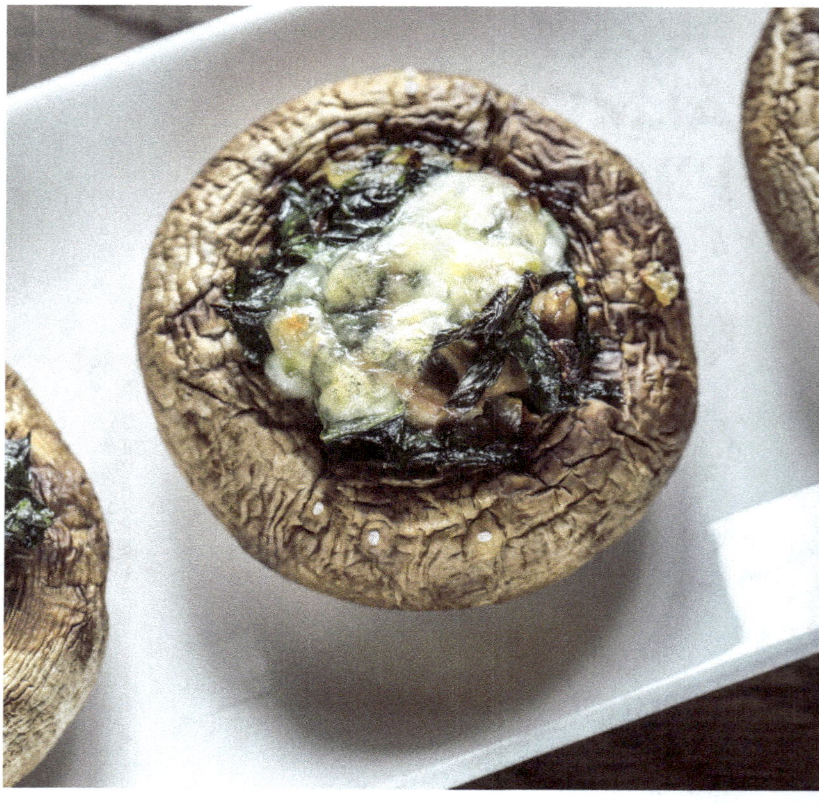

Directions

1. Preheat oven to 375°F (190°C).
2. First, remove the stems from the mushrooms and finely chop them.
3. In a skillet, warm olive oil over moderate heat. Sauté garlic and mushroom stems until softened. Add spinach and cook until wilted.
4. Remove from heat and stir in feta cheese—season with salt and pepper.
5. Fill each mushroom cap with the spinach-feta mixture.
6. Place on a cooking sheet and bake for 20 minutes or until mushrooms are tender.

GREEN PEA AND MINT DIP

Prep time
10 Min

Cook Time
0 Min

Servings
4

Nutrition Information

Calories: 130   Carbs: 14g
Protein: 5g   Fats: 6g

Ingredients

- 2 cups frozen green peas, thawed
- 1/4 cup fresh mint leaves
- 2 tbsp olive oil
- 1 tbsp lemon juice
- Salt and pepper to taste

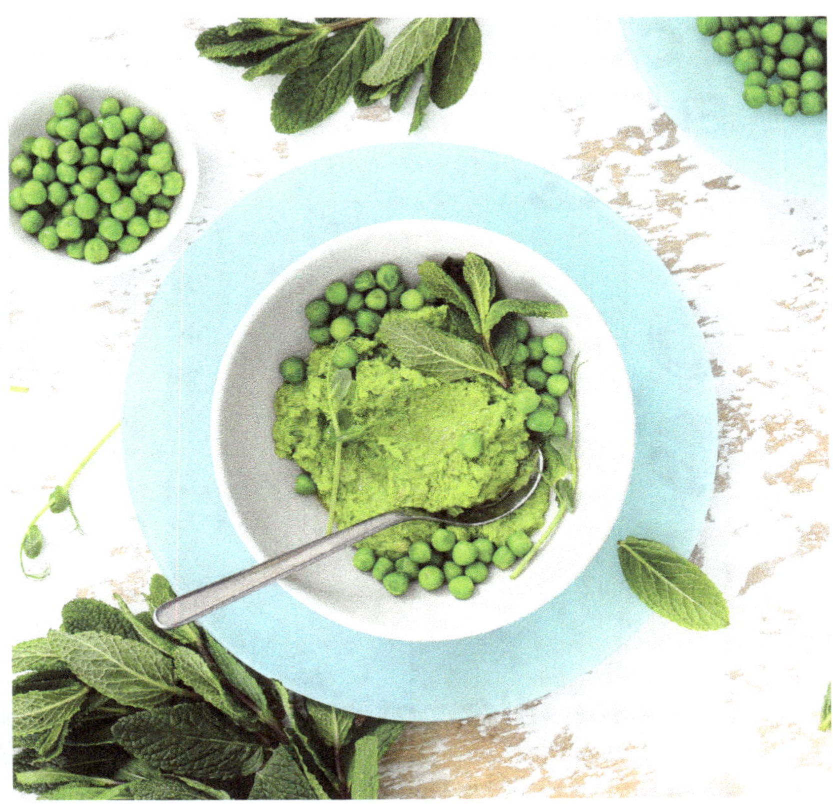

Directions

1. To make the recipe, blend all ingredients into a food processor until they form a smooth mixture.
2. Season with salt and pepper to taste.
3. Serve with vegetable sticks or whole-grain crackers.

COCONUT ENERGY BALLS

Prep time
10 Min

Cook Time
0 Min

Servings
12 Balls

Nutrition Information

Calories: 90   Carbs: 12g
Protein: 2g   Fats: 4g

Ingredients

- 1 cup dates, pitted
- 1/2 cup unsweetened shredded coconut
- 1/2 cup raw almonds
- 1 tbsp chia seeds
- 1 tsp vanilla extract

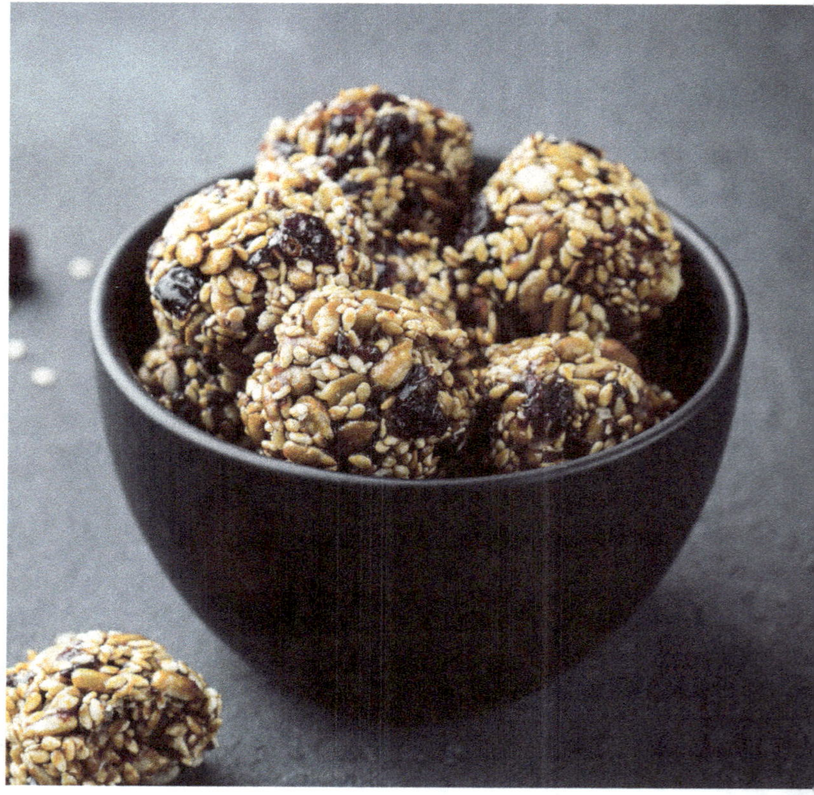

Directions

1. Blend dates, almonds, and vanilla in a food processor until a sticky mixture forms.
2. Add chia seeds and half of the shredded coconut. Pulse a few times to combine.
3. Roll the blending into small balls and coat with the remaining shredded coconut.
4. Refrigerate for about 1 hour before serving.

SESAME SEARED TUNA CUBES

Prep time
10 Min

Cook Time
5 Min

Servings
2

Nutrition Information

Calories: 180   Carbs: 1g
Protein: 25g   Fats: 8g

Ingredients

- 2 tuna steaks (around 1/2 pound total)
- 2 tbsp sesame seeds
- 1 tbsp olive oil
- Salt and pepper to taste
- 2 tbsp soy sauce (for dipping)

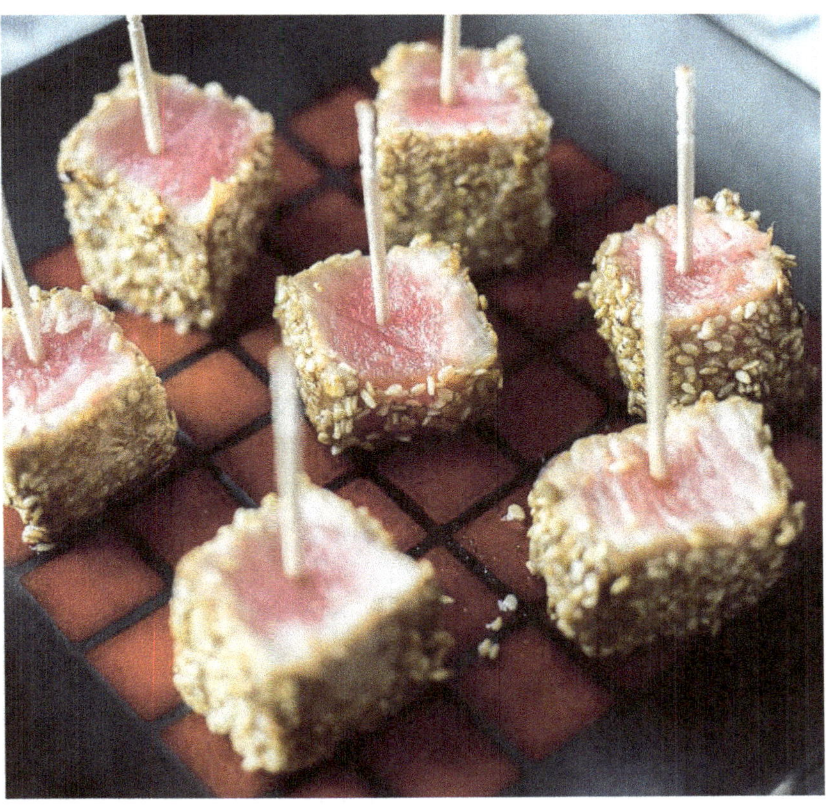

Directions

1. Cut tuna steaks into 1-inch cubes.
2. Season tuna cubes with salt and pepper, then coat all sides with sesame seeds.
3. To cook, warm some olive oil in a skillet on medium-high heat. Sear tuna cubes for about 1 minute on each side.
4. Serve immediately with soy sauce for dipping.

VEGGIE CHIPS WITH AVOCADO DIP

 **Prep time**
15 Min

 **Cook Time**
15 Min

 **Servings**
4

Nutrition Information

Calories: 180   Carbs: 12g
Protein: 3g   Fats: 14g

Ingredients

- 2 zucchinis, thinly sliced
- 2 beets, thinly sliced
- 2 tbsp olive oil
- Salt to taste
- 1 ripe avocado
- Juice of 1 lime
- 1 garlic clove, mince

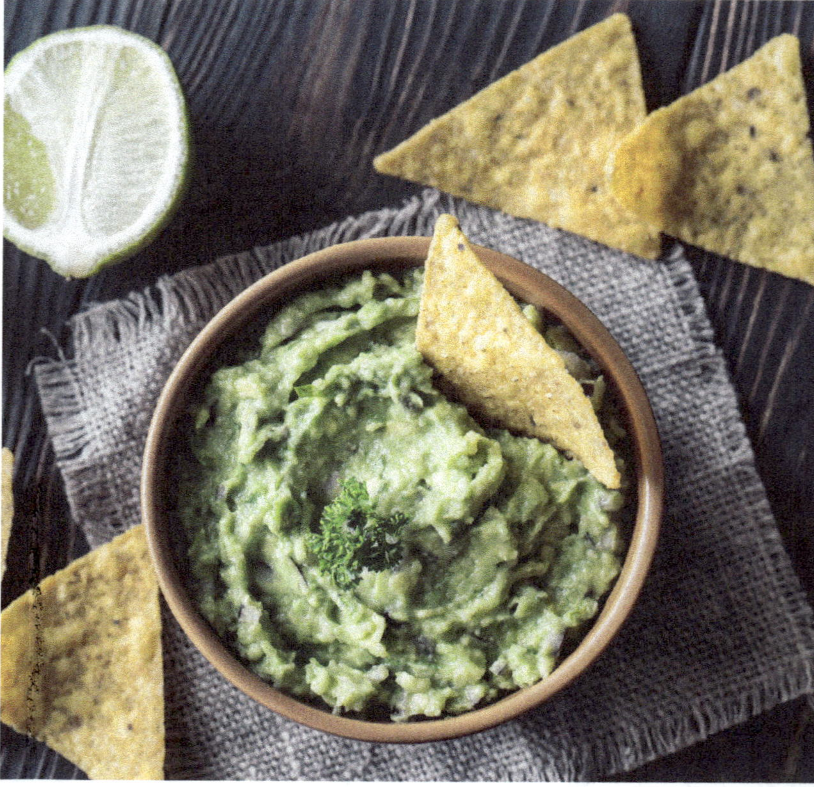

Directions

1. Preheat oven to 375°F (190°C). Toss zucchini and beet slices with olive oil and salt.
2. Arrange the slices on a baking sheet, ensuring they are in a single layer. Bake for 10-15 minutes or until crispy.
3. While the chips are baking, mash the avocado in a bowl. Stir in lime juice and minced garlic.
4. Serve chips with avocado

BROCCOLI AND CHEDDAR BITES

Prep time
15 Min

Cook Time
20 Min

Servings
4

Nutrition Information

Calories: 180

Carbs: 12g

Protein: 10g

Fats: 10g

Ingredients

- 2 cups broccoli florets, steamed and finely chopped
- 1 cup cheddar cheese, shredded
- 2 eggs
- 1/2 cup breadcrumbs
- Salt and pepper to taste

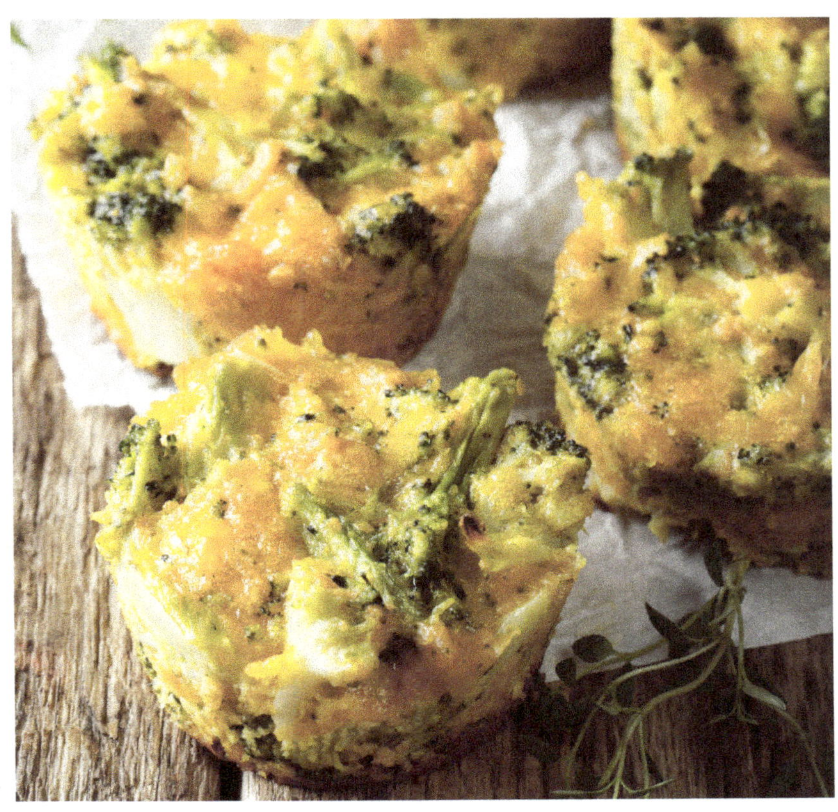

Directions

1. Preheat oven to 375°F (190°C).
2. Combine broccoli, cheddar cheese, eggs, and breadcrumbs in a mixing bowl.
3. Season with salt and pepper.
4. Place the mixture into small balls or patties on a baking sheet.
5. Bake for 20 minutes or until golden and firm.

CARROT STICKS WITH ALMOND BUTTER DIP

 **Prep time**
10 Min

 **Cook Time**
0 Min

 **Servings**
4

Nutrition Information

Calories: 240

Carbs: 18g

Protein: 7g

Fats: 16g

Ingredients

- 4 large carrots, skinned and cut into sticks
- 1/2 cup almond butter
- 1 tbsp honey
- 1 tbsp water

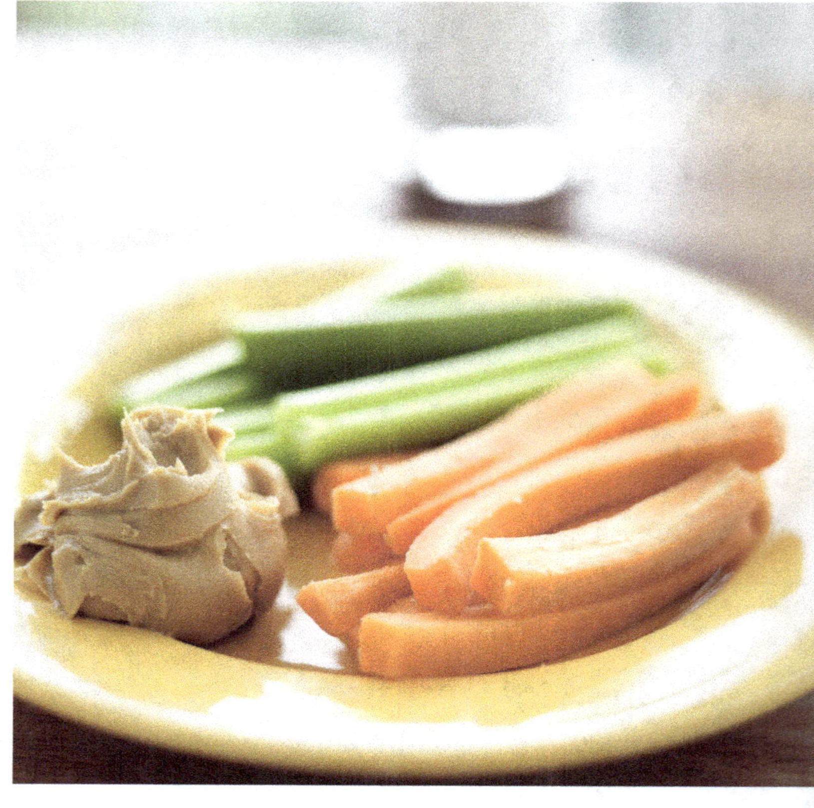

Directions

1. Whisk together almond butter, honey, and water in a small bowl until smooth.
2. Serve carrot sticks with almond butter dip on the side.

SAVORY FLAXSEED CRACKERS

Prep time
15 Min

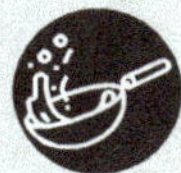

Cook Time
20 Min

Servings
4

Nutrition Information

Calories: 180   Carbs: 8g
Protein: 6g   Fats: 14g

Ingredients

- 1 cup ground flaxseeds
- 1/2 cup water
- 1 tsp Italian seasoning
- 1/4 tsp garlic powder
- Salt to taste

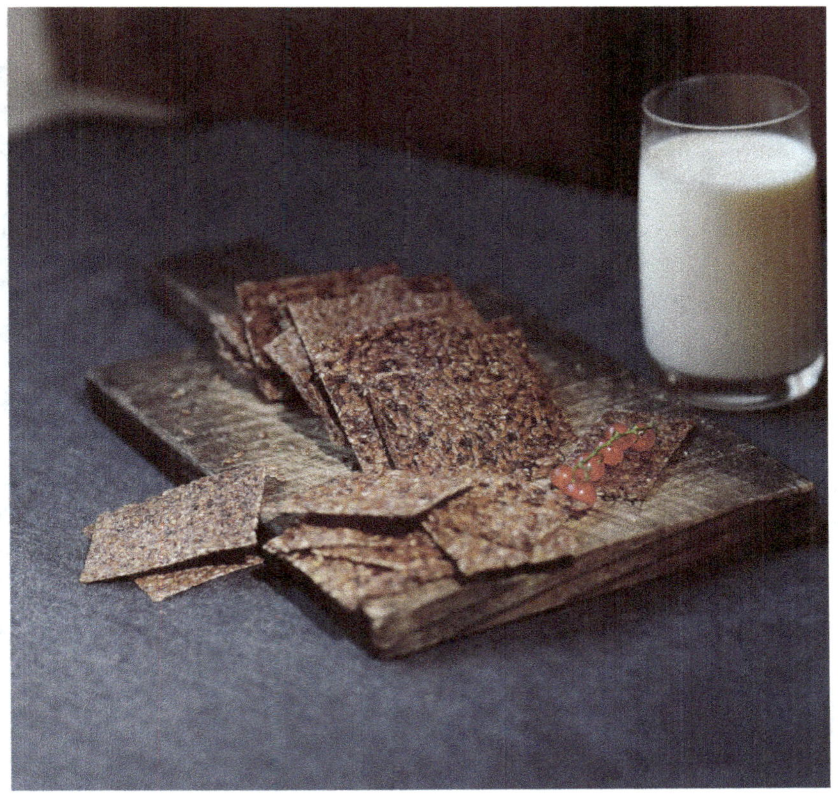

Directions

1. Preheat oven to 350°F (175°C).
2. Mix flaxseeds, water, Italian seasoning, garlic powder, and salt until a dough forms.
3. To make the dough thin, place it between 2 sheets of aluminum foil and roll it out.
4. Cut into cracker shapes using a knife or cookie cutter.
5. Take to a cooking sheet and bake for 20 minutes or until crisp.

MIXED NUTS WITH SEA SALT

Prep time
5 Min

Cook Time
10 Min

Servings
4

Nutrition Information

Calories: 320
Protein: 10g

Carbs: 10g
Fats: 28g

Ingredients

- 2 cups mixed nuts (almonds, cashews, walnuts, etc.)
- 1 tbsp olive oil
- Sea salt to taste

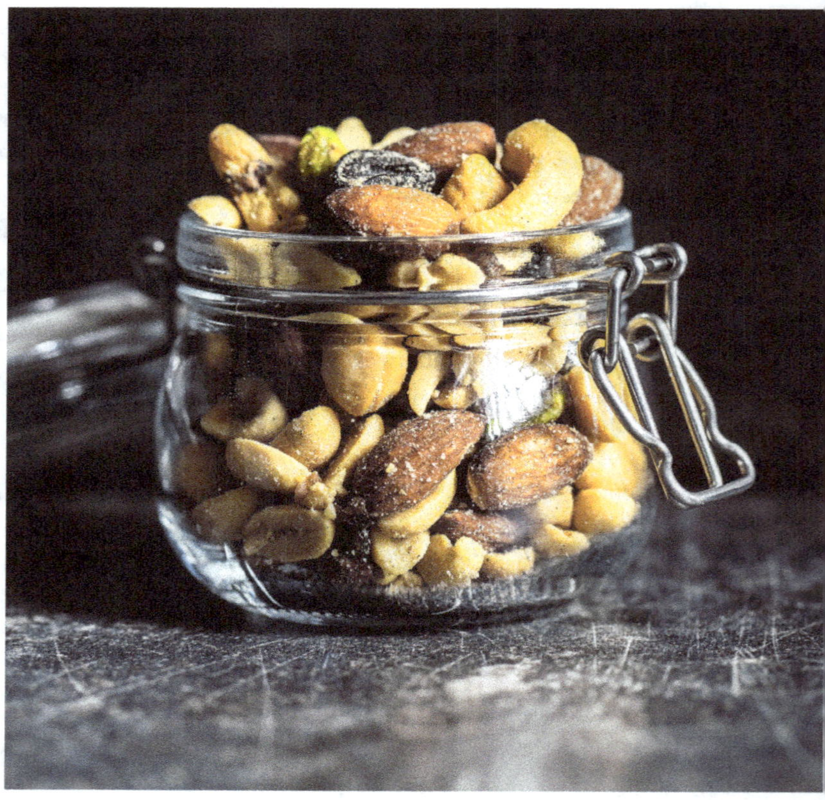

Directions

1. Preheat oven to 350°F (175°C).
2. Toss mixed nuts in olive oil and spread them on a baking sheet.
3. Lightly sprinkle with sea salt.
4. Roast for 10 minutes, stirring halfway.

OLIVE TAPENADE ON CUCUMBER SLICES

Prep time
10 Min

Cook Time
0 Min

Servings
4

Nutrition Information

Calories: 150   Carbs: 4g
Protein: 1g   Fats: 15g

Ingredients

- 1 cup pitted black olives
- 1 garlic clove
- 1 tbsp capers
- 2 tbsp olive oil
- 1 large cucumber, sliced

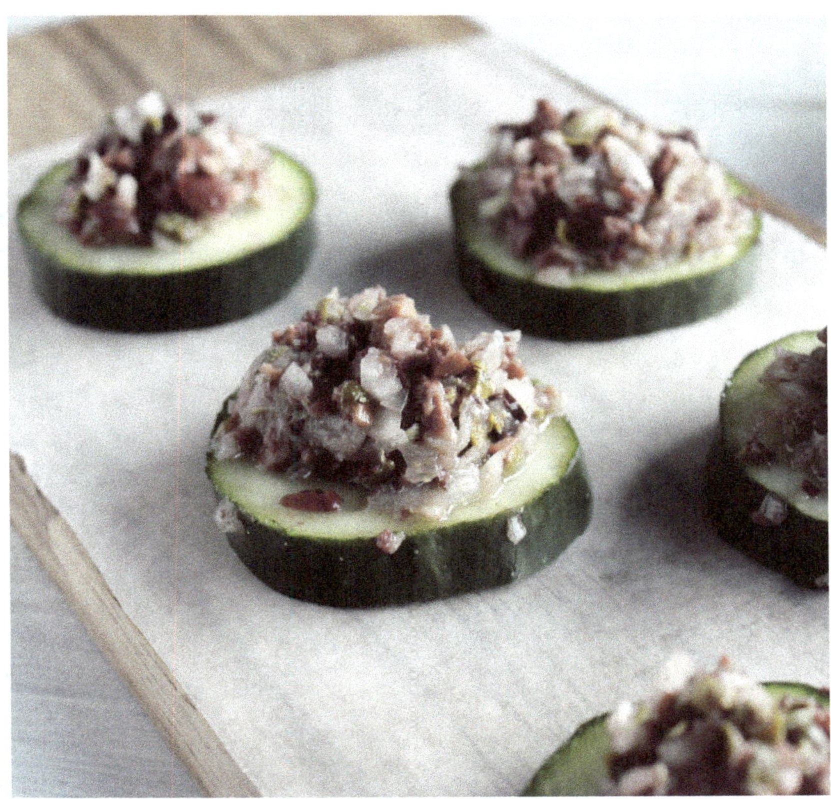

Directions

1. Combine olives, garlic, capers, and olive oil in a food processor. Blend until a coarse paste forms.
2. Place a small dollop of tapenade on each cucumber slice.
3. Serve immediately.

DESSERTS

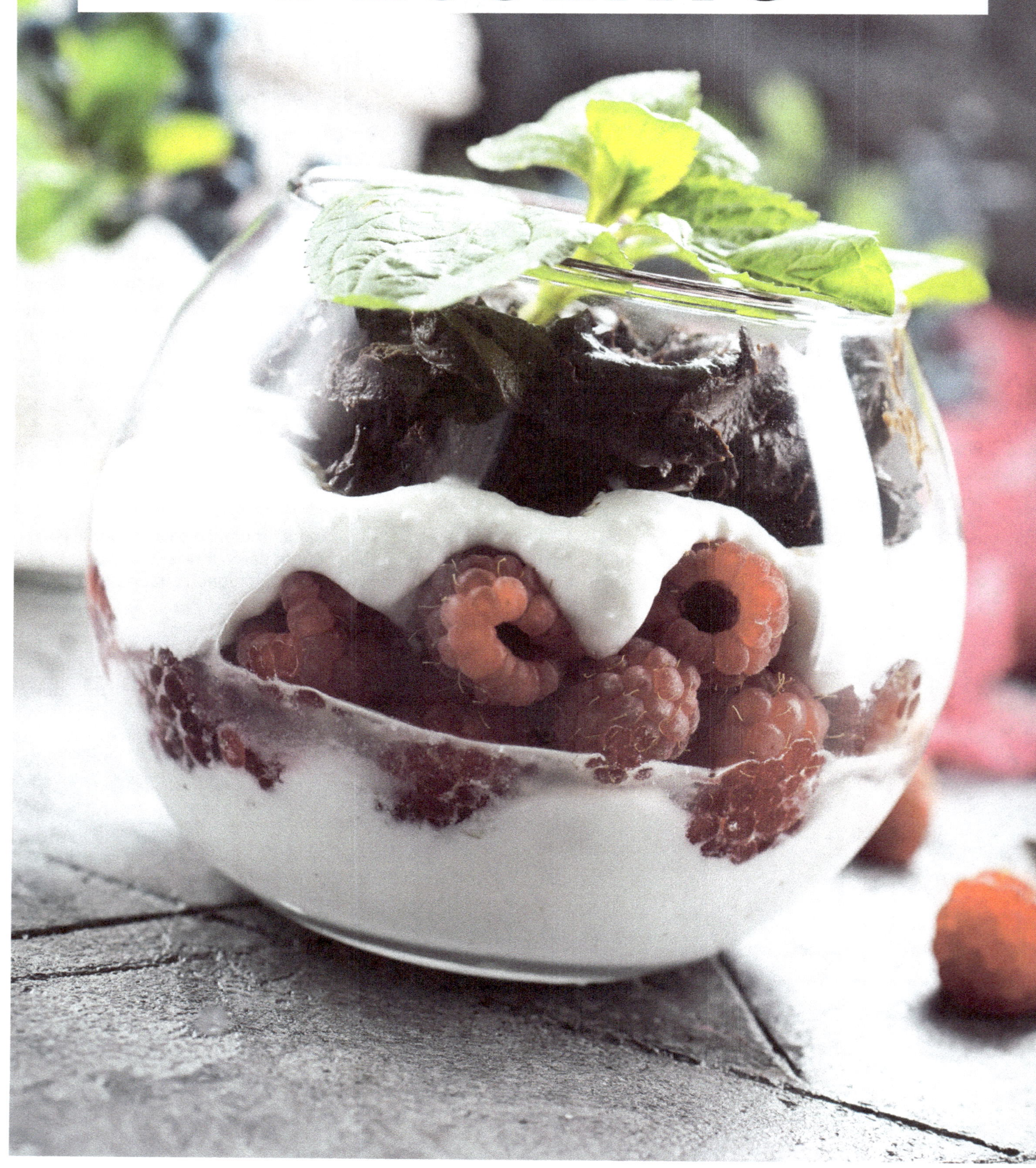

CHOCOLATE AVOCADO MOUSSE

Prep time
10 Min

Cook Time
0 Min

Servings
2

Nutrition Information

Calories: 250   Carbs: 30g
Protein: 3g   Fats: 15g

Ingredients

- 1 ripe avocado, peeled and pitted
- 3 tbsp cocoa powder
- 3 tbsp honey or maple syrup
- 1/2 tsp vanilla extract
- A pinch of salt

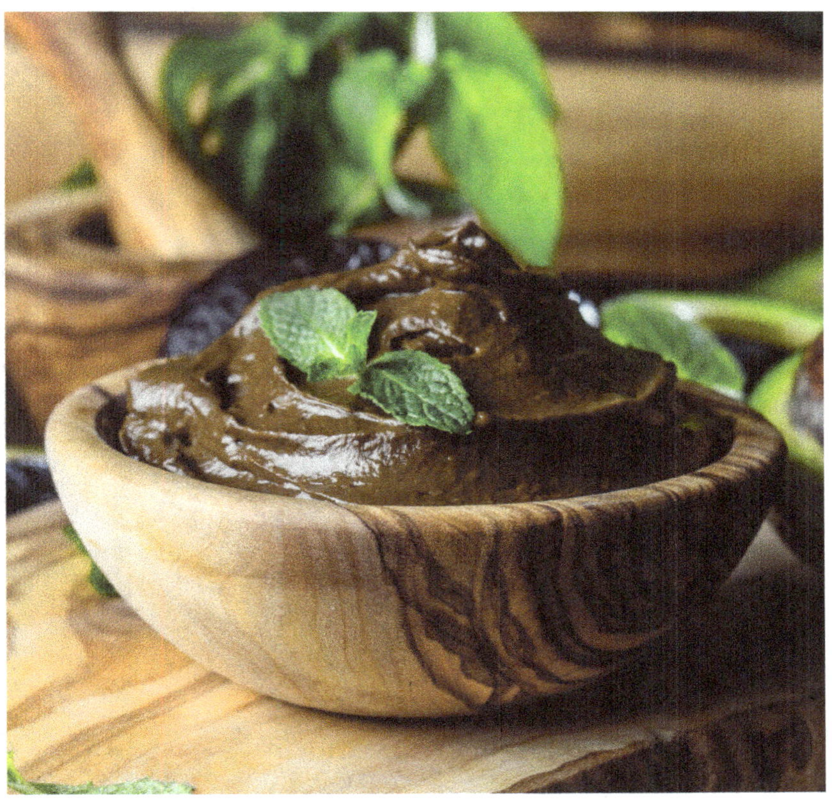

Directions

1. Blend or process all the ingredients until smooth using a blender or food processor.
2. Chill in the refrigerator for at least 2 hours.
3. Serve garnished with some cocoa nibs or fresh berries.

BAKED CINNAMON APPLES

Prep time
10 Min

Cook Time
30 Min

Servings
4

Nutrition Information

Calories: 120   Carbs: 31g
Protein: 1g   Fats: 0.5g

Ingredients

- 4 large apples, cored and sliced
- 2 tsp cinnamon
- 1 tbsp honey or maple syrup
- 1/4 cup water

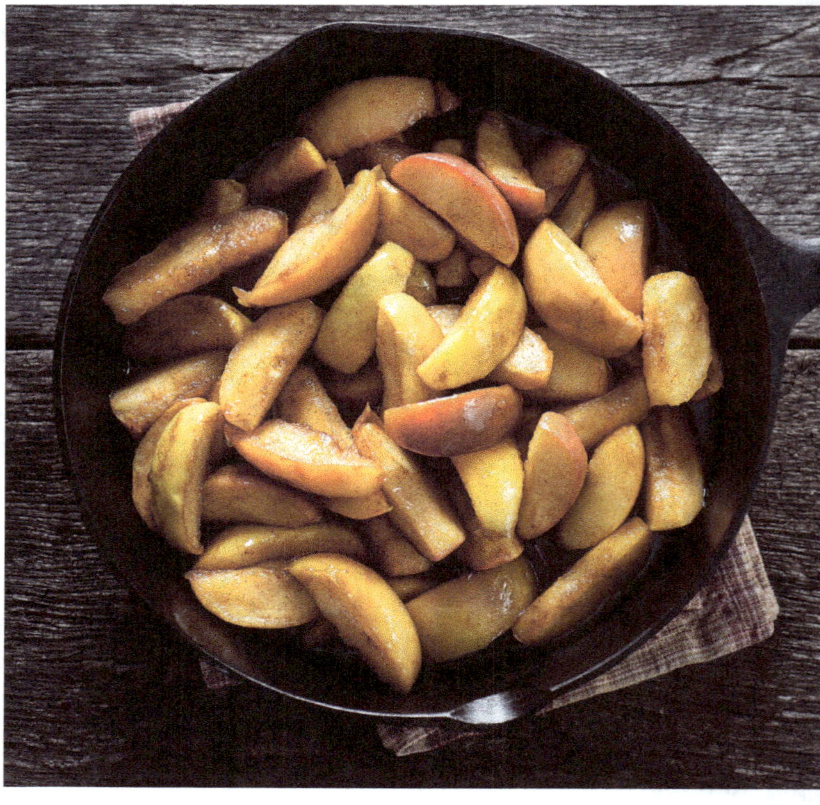

Directions

1. Preheat oven to 350°F (175°C).
2. Place apple slices in a baking dish.
3. Drink maple syrup into your plate and sprinkle it with cinnamon for extra sweetness and flavor.
4. Pour water into the container.
5. Prepare for 30 minutes or until the apples are soft.
6. Serve warm.

COCONUT AND ALMOND TRUFFLES

Prep time
15 Min

Cook Time
0 Min

Servings
6

Nutrition Information

Calories: 220
Protein: 5g

Carbs: 12g
Fats: 18g

Ingredients

- 1 cup shredded coconut, unsweetened
- 1/2 cup almond butter
- 2 tbsp honey
- 1/4 tsp vanilla extract
- A pinch of salt
- 1/4 cup almonds, chopped for coating

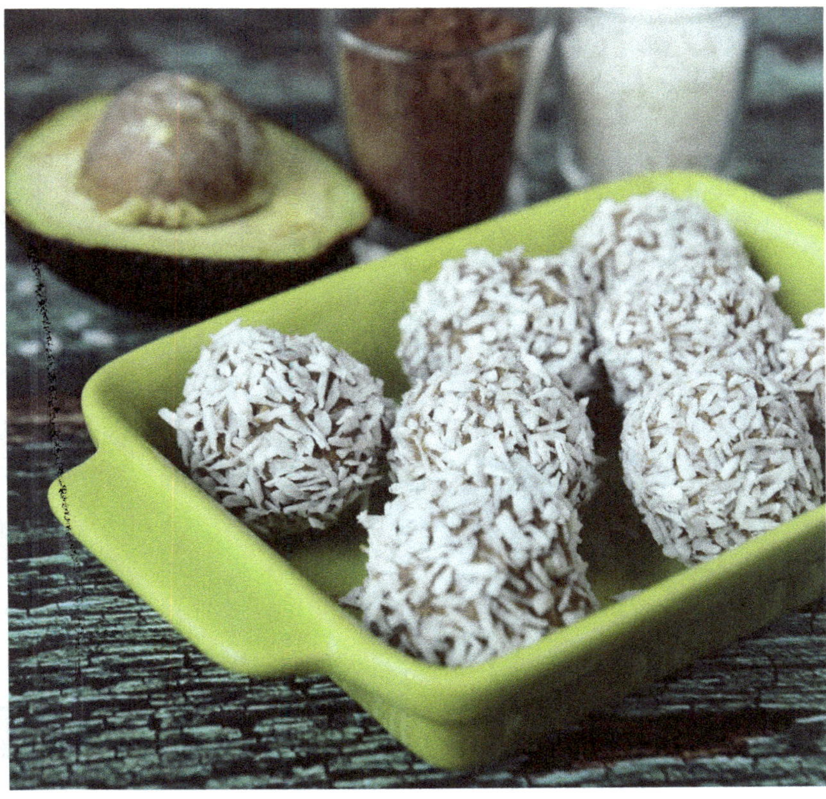

Directions

1. Combine shredded coconut, almond butter, honey, vanilla, and salt in a mixing bowl.
2. Shape the mixture into small balls.
3. Roll each truffle in the chopped almonds to coat.
4. Place in the refrigerator for at least 1 hour to set.

DARK CHOCOLATE DIPPED STRAWBERRIES

Prep time
10 Min

Cook Time
5 Min

Servings
4

Nutrition Information

Calories: 140

Carbs: 15g

Protein: 2g

Fats: 8g

Ingredients

- 12 large strawberries, washed and dried
- 100g dark chocolate (at least 70% cocoa)
- 1 tsp coconut oil

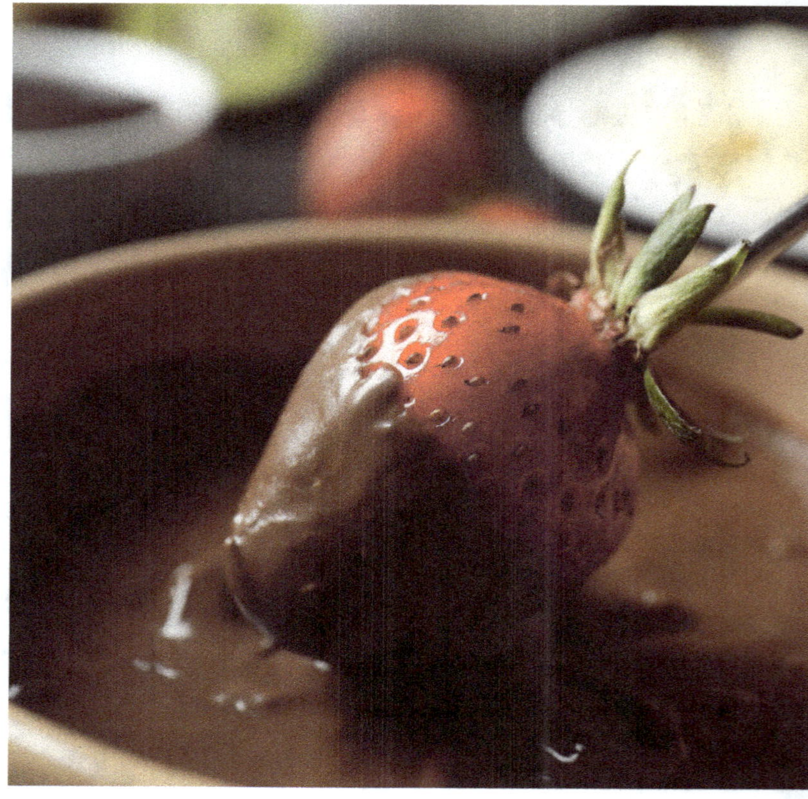

Directions

1. To melt the dark chocolate and coconut oil, kindly place them in a heat-proof bowl and heat them over a pan of simmering water or microwave.
2. Use each strawberry and dip it into the melted chocolate, ensuring it is fully coated.
3. Place on parchment paper and let cool. Chill in the refrigerator for 30 minutes to set.

RASPBERRY AND CHIA SEED PUDDING

Prep time
10 Min

Cook Time
0 Min

Servings
4

Nutrition Information

Calories: 120
Protein: 4g

Carbs: 15g
Fats: 5g

Ingredients

- 1/4 cup chia seeds
- 1 cup almond milk
- 1/2 cup raspberries (plus some for garnish)
- 1 tbsp honey or maple syrup

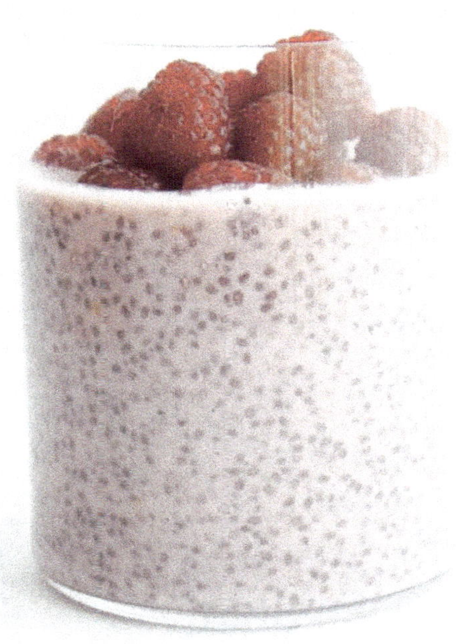

Directions

1. Mash raspberries in a bowl.
2. Add chia seeds, almond milk, and honey. Mix well.
3. Transfer to serving glasses and refrigerate overnight or at least 4 hours.
4. Garnish with fresh raspberries before serving.

LEMON AND COCONUT BLISS BALLS

Prep time
15 Min

Cook Time
0 Min

Servings
8

Nutrition Information

Calories: 140   Carbs: 12g
Protein: 2g   Fats: 9g

Ingredients

- 1 cup unsweetened shredded coconut
- Zest and juice of 1 lemon
- 1/2 cup cashews, absorbed in water for 2 hours
- 2 tbsp honey or maple syrup
- A pinch of salt

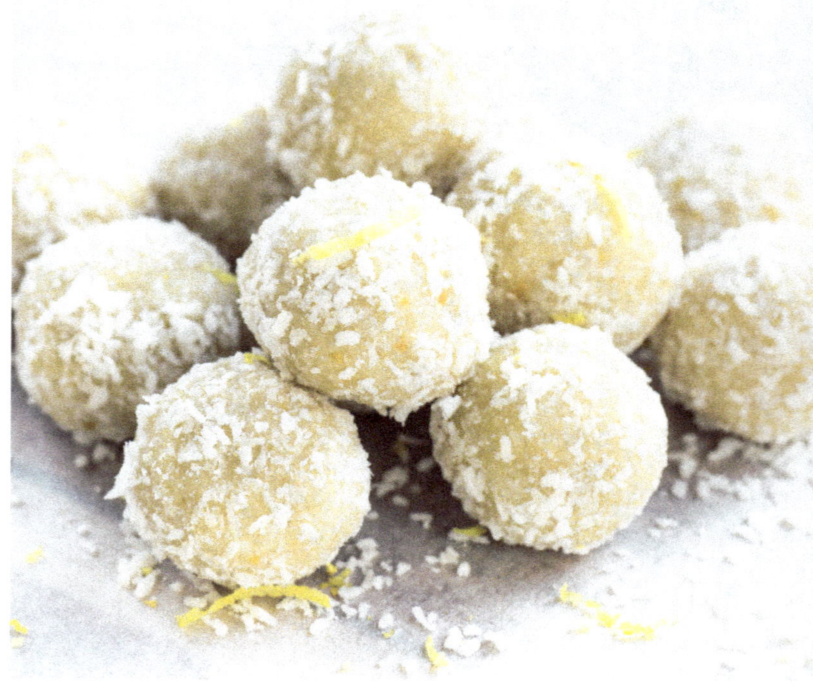

Directions

1. In a food processor, blend soaked cashews until smooth.
2. Add shredded coconut, lemon zest, lemon juice, honey, and salt. Process until the mixture forms a dough.
3. Roll into balls and refrigerate for at least 1 hour before serving.

SUGAR-FREE PUMPKIN PIE

Prep time
15 Min

Cook Time
45 Min

Servings
8

Nutrition Information

Calories: 180   Carbs: 20g
Protein: 5g   Fats: 10g

Ingredients

- 1 prepared pie crust (gluten-free optional)
- 1 can (15 oz) pumpkin puree
- 3 eggs
- 1/4 cup almond milk
- 1 tsp vanilla extract
- 1/4 cup erythritol or another sugar substitute
- 2 tsp pumpkin pie spice

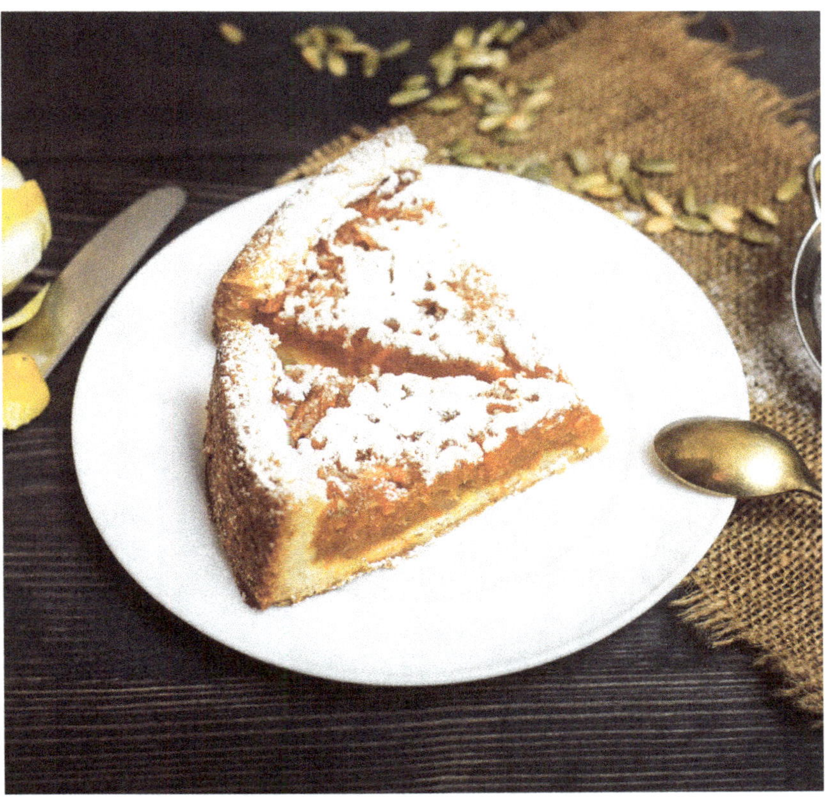

Directions

1. Preheat oven to 350°F (175°C).
2. Whisk together pumpkin puree, eggs, almond milk, vanilla, erythritol, and pumpkin pie spice in a mixing bowl.
3. Pour the blending into the prepared pie crust.
4. Bake for 45 minutes or until the center is set.
5. Allow to cool and refrigerate for a few hours before serving.

WALNUT AND DATE BROWNIES

Prep time
15 Min

Cook Time
20 Min

Servings
12

Nutrition Information

Calories: 150   Carbs: 18g
Protein: 3g   Fats: 9g

Ingredients

- 1 cup dates, pitted
- 1 cup walnuts
- 1/4 cup cocoa powder
- 1 tsp vanilla extract
- A pinch of salt

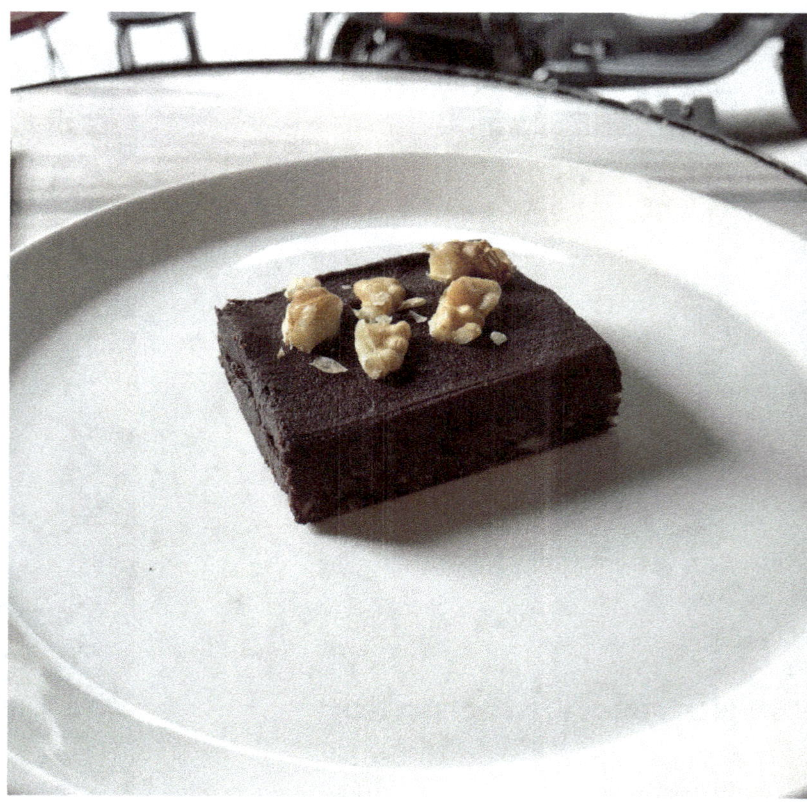

Directions

1. Preheat oven to 350°F (175°C).
2. Blend dates and walnuts in a blend processor until they form a dough.
3. Mix cocoa powder, vanilla, and salt in the blender until thoroughly incorporated.
4. Press the mixture into a lined brownie pan.
5. Bake for 20 minutes.
6. Cool and cut into squares.

ALMOND JOY ENERGY BITES

Prep time
15 Min

Cook Time
0 Min

Servings
8

Nutrition Information

Calories: 110   Carbs: 8g
Protein: 3g   Fats: 8g

Ingredients

- 1/2 cup almonds, soaked for 2 hours
- 1/4 cup unsweetened shredded coconut
- 2 tbsp cocoa powder
- 2 tbsp honey or maple syrup

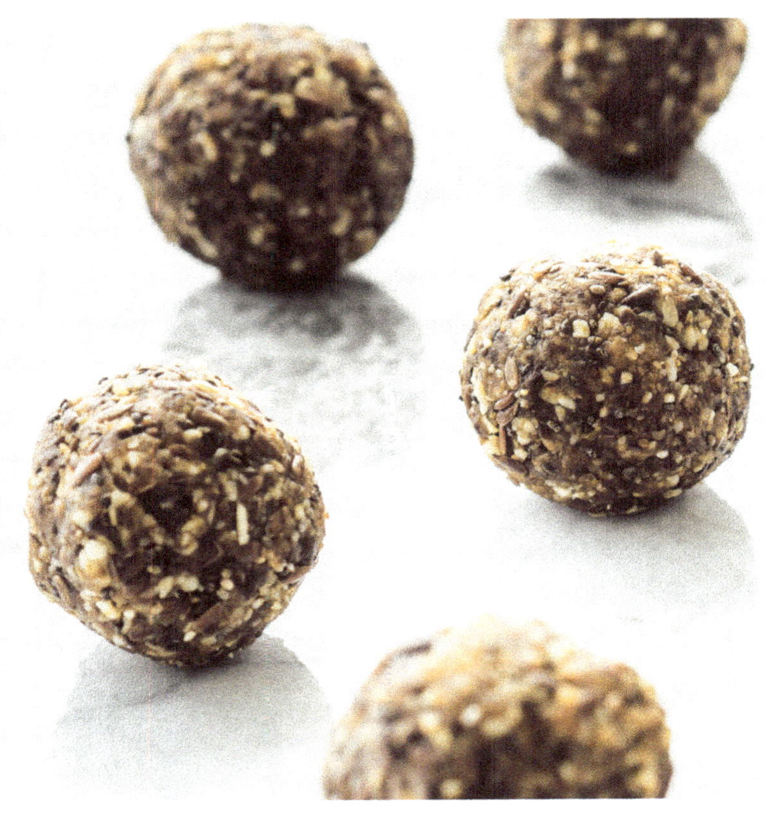

Directions

1. Blend almonds in a food processor until they're finely ground.
2. Add shredded coconut, cocoa powder, and honey. Blend until the mixture forms a dough.
3. Roll into balls and refrigerate for at least 1 hour before serving.

COCONUT CREAM & MIXED BERRY PARFAIT

Prep time
10 Min

Cook Time
0 Min

Servings
4

Nutrition Information

Calories: 240

Carbs: 20g

Protein: 2g

Fats: 18g

Ingredients

- 1 can (14 oz) full-fat coconut milk, chilled overnight
- 1 cup mixed berries (blueberries, raspberries, strawberries)
- 2 tbsp honey or maple syrup
- 1/2 tsp vanilla extract

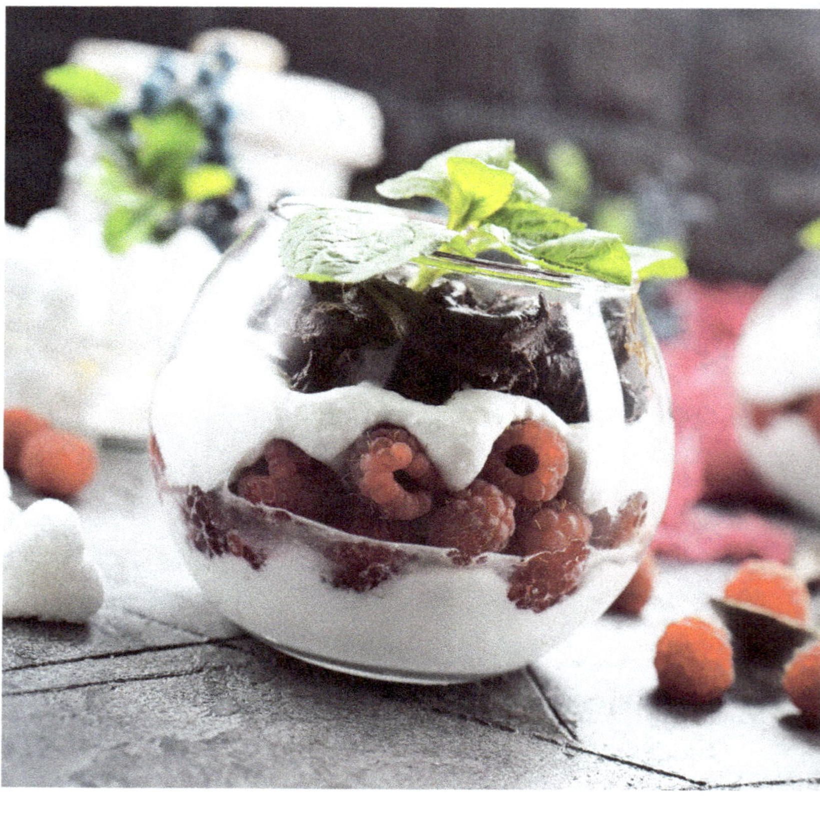

Directions

1. Transfer the thick coconut cream from the top of the can into a separate bowl.
2. Add vanilla and honey, and whip until creamy.
3. Layer coconut cream and mixed berries in serving glasses, starting and ending with coconut cream.
4. Top with a few more berries and serve chilled.